ADVANCED TOPICS
IN SCIENCE AND TECHNOLOGY IN CHINA

ADVANCED TOPICS IN SCIENCE AND TECHNOLOGY IN CHINA

Zhejiang University is one of the leading universities in China. In Advanced Topics in Science and Technology in China, Zhejiang University Press and Springer jointly publish monographs by Chinese scholars and professors, as well as invited authors and editors from abroad who are outstanding experts and scholars in their fields. This series will be of interest to researchers, lecturers, and graduate students alike.

Advanced Topics in Science and Technology in China aims to present the latest and most cutting-edge theories, techniques, and methodologies in various research areas in China. It covers all disciplines in the fields of natural science and technology, including but not limited to, computer science, materials science, life sciences, engineering, environmental sciences, mathematics, and physics.

Jian'an Wang
Xiaojie Xie
(Editors)

Mesenchymal Stem Cells for the Heart
From Bench to Bedside

With 10 figures

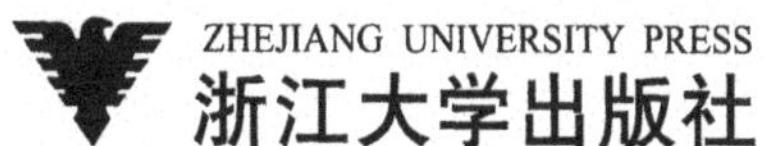

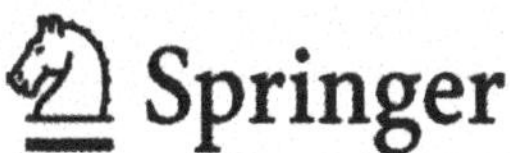

EDITORS:

Prof. Jian'an Wang
Second Affiliated Hospital,
Zhejiang University College of Medicine,
Hangzhou 310008, China
E-mail: wja@zju.edu.cn

Dr. Xiaojie Xie
Second Affiliated Hospital,
Zhejiang University College of Medicine,
Hangzhou 310008, China
E-mail: xiaojiexie@hotmail.com

ISBN 978-7-308-06167-4 **Zhejiang University Press, Hangzhou**
ISBN 978-3-540-88149-0 **Springer Berlin Heidelberg New York**
e-ISBN 978-3-540-88150-6 **Springer Berlin Heidelberg New York**

Series ISSN 1995-6819 Advanced topics in science and technology in China
Series e-ISSN 1995-6827 Advanced topics in science and technology in China

Library of Congress Control Number: 2008936092

Co-published by Zhejiang University Press, Hangzhou and Springer-Verlag GmbH Berlin Heidelberg

Springer is a part of Springer Science+Business Media
springer.com

Cover design: Frido Steinen-Broo, EStudio Calamar, Spain
Printed on acid-free paper

Preface

With the aging of the population worldwide, ischemic heart disease remains a leading cause of morbidity and mortality in China and western countries despite substantial advances in risk factor control, drug therapy and revascularization therapy. Cell therapy is currently being investigated as an additional treatment for patients with ischemic heart disease. Favorable results obtained in preclinical studies have led to a rapid introduction of cardiac cell therapy in clinical trials. It has been demonstrated that mesenchymal stem cells (MSCs) are available for tissue engineering and therapeutic applications because of their multipotent differentiation and relative ease of isolation from adult tissues. The therapeutic effects of MSCs on myocardial repair may be due to multiple factors, including transdifferentiation into cardiac cells, varieties of paracrine cytokines and growth factors promoting neoangiogenesis and attenuating apoptosis, spontaneous cell fusion and initiation of endogenous repair mechanisms, etc.

Although inspiring results have been obtained in several studies, the therapeutic effects and exact mechanisms of MSCs on clinical patients suffering from heart disease remain to be further clarified. However, a series of studies indicate that the application of MSCs might be associated with some cardiac risks as well, including differentiation into unwanted mesenchymal cell types, the occurrence of cytogenetic instability upon prolonged expansion, etc. The discrepancies observed in clinical trials necessitate definitive validation prior to *in vivo* application.

This book intends to give us a comprehensive look at MSCs from both the viewpoint of basic research to clinical investigations, presenting the pros and cons of MSC therapy for ischemic heart disease, highlighting recent discoveries in MSCs biological and immunological characteristics, multilineage transdifferentiation and utilization in cardiac repair, current status in clinical application, etc. We hope this book will be helpful for both researchers and cardiologists engaged in stem cell researches. You are welcome to share your opinions with us and discuss any problem in this book.

Jian-an Wang

Contents

1

MSCs Isolation and Culture *Ex Vivo*

Xiaojie Xie[1], Chun Gui[2]

[1]Second Affiliated Hospital, Zhejiang University College of Medicine, Hangzhou,China
E-mail: xiaojiexie@hotmail.com
[2]First Affiliated Hospital, Guangxi Medical University, Guilin,China
E-mail: gui_chun@126.com

Abstract: Mesenchymal stem cells (MSCs) can almost be found in any adult organ. They can be isolated and expanded within several weeks up to hundreds of millions of cells. The cell isolation based on the surface antigen expression may significantly enrich for the desired cell population and reduce the time required for cell expansion. This chapter aims to introduce the isolation and *ex vivo* culture method of MSCs widely used in China, including direct adherence, density gradient centrifugation and magnetic microbead or flow cytometry. To keep cell lines and store cells for later use, this chapter also introduces MSCs cryopreservation and thawing procedures.

Mesenchymal stem cells (MSCs), also named as mesenchymal progenitor cells, are self-renewable and multipotent stem cells that can differentiate into a variety of cell types. It has been demonstrated that MSCs can differentiate *in vitro* or *in vivo* into some lineage cells (Pittenger et al, 1999), including osteoblasts (Sila-Asna et al, 2007; Friedman et al, 2006), chondrocytes (Bernardo et al, 2007), myocytes (Toma et al, 2002), adipocytes (Sanchez-Ramos et al, 2000) and neurocytes (Sanchez-Ramos et al, 2000). Classically,

MSCs have been obtained from the bone marrow, sometimes referred to as marrow stromal cells (Campagnoli et al, 2001; Erices et al, 2000; Lee et al, 2004; Suva et al, 2004). While the terms, mesenchymal stem cell and stromal cell have been used interchangeably, they are now increasingly recognized as separate entities. Stromal cells are a highly heterogenous cell population consisting of multiple cell types with differing potential for proliferation and differentiation. In contrast, MSCs represent a more homogenous sub-population of mononuclear progenitor cells possessing stem cell features and specific cell surface markers. McCulloch and Till first revealed the clonal nature of marrow cells in the 1960s (Becker et al, 1963; Siminovitch et al, 1963). An *ex vivo* assay for examining the clonogenic potential of multipotent marrow cells was later reported in the 1970s by Friedenstein and colleagues (Friedenstein, 1966, 1974). In this assay system, stromal cells were referred to as colony-forming unit-fibroblasts (CFU-f).

MSCs can be derived from other non-marrow tissues, such as the liver and adipose, as well as amniotic fluid and umbilical cord blood (Campagnoli et al, 2001; Erices et al, 2000; Lee et al, 2004). MSCs comprise 0.001%~0.1% of the total population of marrow nucleated cells, and can be expanded *in vitro* extensively without loss of function or phenotype (Pittenger et al, 1999; Gerson, 1999). Neither hematopoietic surface molecules (CD34, CD45, and CD14) nor endothelial markers (CD34, CD31, and vWF) are detectable on the cellular membrane of MSCs (Prockop, 1997; Majumdar et al, 1998). MSCs are recognized as expressing a large number of polyglucoproteins, such as intercellular adhesion molecules (CD44, CD29, CD90), stromal cell markers (SH-2, SH-3, SH-4) and cytokine receptors [interleukin-1 (IL-1) receptor, tumor necrosis factor-alpha (TNF-α) receptor] (Majumdar et al, 1998). Techniques are now available to isolate bone-marrow-derived mononuclear cells and expand the purified MSCs *ex vivo* in some conditions without change of phenotype or loss of function.

1.1 Cell Isolation

Technically, MSCs are isolated from bone marrow mononuclear cells and separated from hematopoietic stem cells on the basis of their selective adherence to the culture surface. The suspended cells, consisting of hematpoietic stem cells, are removed by changing the medium. According to the different density of bone marrow cells, MSCs can be aspirated by gradient centrifugation on Percoll (density 1.073 g ml^{-1}) or Ficoll-Hypaque (1.077 g ml^{-1}). With further investigation of surface markers on MSCs, it is possible to isolate MSCs by microbeads with fluorescence-activated cell sorting (FACS) or magnetic-activated cell sorting (MACS). Cells are sorted out with negative expression of endothelial and hematopoietic cell markers and incubated as the primary cultures. By contrast, MSCs express a large number of adhesion molecules and stromal cell markers, allowing for positive sorting by microbeads. This procedure requires advanced techniques and can be expensive. Therefore, we would like to introduce an alternative culture method widely used in China (Xie et al, 2006; Huang et al, 2007; Niu et al, 2004).

1.1.1 Direct Adherence Method

1.1.1.1 Materials

Dubelcco's modified Eagle's medium (DMEM) supplemented with 100 U ml^{-1} penicillin G and 100 U ml^{-1} streptomycin; fetal bovine serum (FBS, Gibco) incubated at 56 ℃ inactivate compliments (some investigators think heat-inactivation is unnecessary); sterile phosphate buffered solution (PBS), heparin, etc.

1.1.1.2 Procedures

For human MSCs isolation, 50 ml of human bone marrow is obtained from the donor's iliac crest, diluted at a ratio of 1:1 with DMEM containing heparin (100 U ml^{-1}). After centrifugation at a rate of 1,000 rpm at 4 ℃ for about 10 minutes, bone marrow cells are harvested and resuspended with DMEM supplemented with 10% FBS. Cells are seeded on a culture plate or in a flask at a density of 5×10^7 ml^{-1}, and incubated at 37 ℃ in humid air with 5% CO_2.

For rat or mouse MSCs, animals are sacrificed, femurae and tibiae dissected, and the proximal and distal ends removed. The medullar cavity is opened and rinsed via a syringe with DMEM or PBS containing heparin. The diluted marrow is harvested and then centrifuged at a rate of 1,000 rpm at 4 ℃ for about 10 minutes. Cells are seeded on a culture plate or in a flask at a density of 5×10^7 ml^{-1}, and incubated at 37 ℃ in humid air with 5% CO_2.

The medium should be changed to remove non-adherent cells at 24~48 h after primary seeding, and every 4 to 5 days thereafter. Once primary cells grow to cover over 80% to 90% of the culture surface, cells are passaged onto a new plate or into a new flask.

In some laboratories this direct adherence method is employed to isolate MSCs. One unavoidable disadvantage of this method is that the cultured MSCs can be contaminated with non-MSCs, such as hematopoietic stem cells, progenitor endothelial cells, etc. Thus, another method, density gradient centrifugation, may be necessary to separate MSCs.

1.1.2 Density Gradient Centrifugation

This technique also uses Percoll or Ficoll-Hypaque, which are registered trademarks owned by GE Healthcare companies.

Percoll is used for the isolation of cells, organelles and viruses using density centrifugation. Percoll consists of colloidal silica particles of 15~30 nm diameters (23% w/w in water), which have been coated with polyvinylpyrrolidone (PVP) (Laurent, 1980a, 1980b; Laurent and Pertoft, 1980). The PVP coating renders the product completely non-toxic and is ideal for use with biological materials. The PVP is firmly bound to the silica particles as a monomolecular layer. Due to its heterogeneity in particle size, sedimentation occurs at different rates, spontaneously creating very smooth, isometric gradients in the range of 1.0~1.3 g ml^{-1}. Percoll is best used in balanced salt solutions, sterile saline or 0.25 M sucrose. Cells can be separated in gradients in balanced salts solutions. It is recommended that the separation of most biological particles be carried out in Percoll diluted with sucrose (0.25 M final concentration). The low osmolarity of Percoll permits this parameter to be controlled by the user without interference from the density medium itself. The addition of 9 parts (v/v) of Percoll to one part (v/v) of either 1.5 M NaCl, 10 × concentrated culture medium or 2.5 M sucrose will result in a solution adjusted to approximately 340 mOsm/kg·H_2O. Final adjustments can be made with the addition of salts or distilled water. The precise osmolarity should be checked prior to using with an osmometer. Living cells can be separated from the Percoll medium by washing with sterile saline [5 parts (v/v) to 1 part (v/v) of cell suspension]. The washing may be repeated two to three times and the cells collected between each washing step by centrifugation at 400 g for 5~10 minutes.

Ficoll is a neutral, highly branched, high-mass, hydrophilic polysaccharide which dissolves readily in aqueous solutions (Abildgaard, 1996). Ficoll radii range from 2~7 nm. Ficoll is prepared by reaction of the polysaccharide with epichlorohydrin. Ficoll is part of Ficoll-Hypaque that is used in biology laboratories to separate blood into its components (erythrocytes, leukocytes, etc). Ficoll-Hypaque is normally placed at the bottom of a column, and blood is then slowly layered above Ficoll-Hypaque. After being centrifuged, the following layers will be visible in the column, from top to bottom: plasma and other constituents, mononuclear cells (PBMC/MNC), Ficoll-Hypaque, erythrocytes and granulocytes which should be present in pellet form. This separation allows an easy harvest of mononuclear cells. It should be noted that some red blood cells trapping (presence of erythrocytes & granulocytes) might occur in the PBMC or Ficoll-Hypaque layer. Major blood clotting may sometimes occur in the PBMC layer. Ethylene diamine tetra-acetate (EDTA) is commonly used in conjunction with Ficoll-Hypaque to prevent clotting.

1.1.2.1 Materials

Dubelcco's modified Eagle's medium (DMEM) supplemented with 100 U ml^{-1} penicillin G and 100 U ml^{-1} streptomycin; fetal bovine serum (FBS, Gibco) incubated at 56 ℃ to inactivate compliments; sterile phosphate buffered solution (PBS); Percoll (density 1.073 g ml^{-1}) or Ficoll-Hypaque (density 1.077 g ml^{-1}); EDTA (ethylene diamine tetra-acetate) or heparin, etc. (Fig. 1.1).

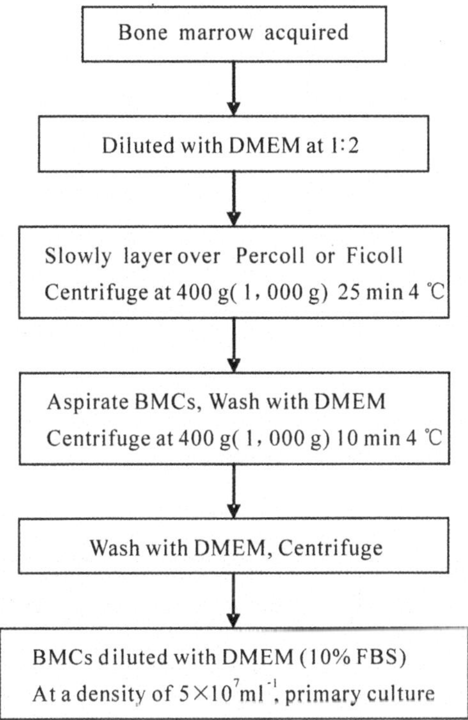

Fig. 1.1. Isolation of MSCs using density gradient centrifugation

1.1.2.2 Procedures

For human MSCs culture, 50 ml of human bone marrow is obtained from the donor's iliac crest, diluted with DMEM containing EDTA or heparin at a ratio of 1:2, and slowly layered above an equal volume of Percoll (1.073 g ml^{-1}) or Ficoll (1.077 g ml^{-1}) solution. For rat or mouse MSCs, animals are sacrificed, femurae and tibiae dissected, the proximal and distal ends removed. The medullar cavity is opened and rinsed via a syringe with DMEM or PBS contained EDTA. The diluted marrow is harvested and then slowly layered above Percoll or Ficoll-Hypaque. The centrifugation rate is 400 g for Percoll, while 1,000 g should be used for Ficoll-Hypaque.

After centrifuging at 4 ℃ for about 25 min, bone marrow-derived mononuclear cells (BMCs) are separated over the gradient interface and are visible in white (Fig. 1.2). BMCs are aspirated and diluted with DMEM. The washing may be repeated two to three times and the cells are collected between each washing step by centrifugation at 400 g for 10 minutes. BMCs are seeded on a culture plate or flask at a density of 5×10^7 ml^{-1}, and incubated with DMEM containing 10% FBS at 37 ℃ in humid air with 5% CO_2.

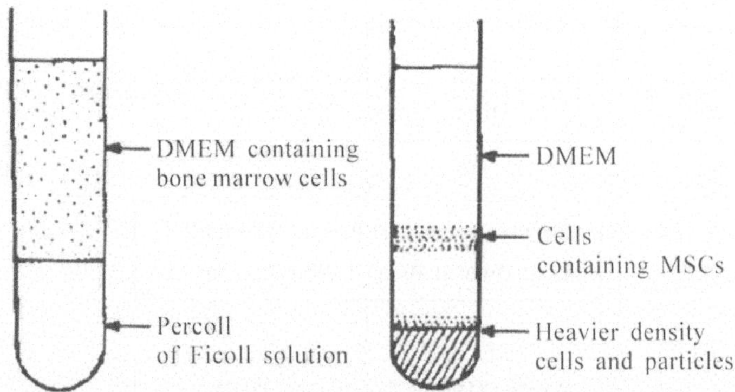

Fig. 1.2. Separated BMCs using Percoll or Ficoll-Hypaque

The medium should be changed to remove non-adherent cells at 24~48 h after primary seeding, and every 4 to 5 days thereafter. Once primary cells grow over 80% to 90% of the culture surface, cells are passaged onto a new plate or into a new flask.

When using Percolll or Ficoll-Hypaque, the dilution of BMCs by DMEM depends on the isolated cells, including the original tissue, as well as the number and the size of cells. When diluting, the appropriate volume of DMEM to a certain cell density of unseparated bone marrow can guarantee the result of the isolation procedures. BMCs isolation by both Percoll and Ficoll-Hypaque is efficient, but the purity and viability of acquired cells can differ. Separated cells are purer when using Percoll, while the biological viability of isolated cells is much better using Ficoll-Hypaque. By contrast, cells acquired by the direct adherence method are not uniform, but their ability for multipotential differentiation and proliferation is improved. Although isolation by density gradient centrifugation allows for more uniformity, the isolated cells' ability for multipotential differentiation and proliferation is diminished.

1.1.3 Magnetic Microbead or Flow Cytometry Method

MSCs have a positive expression of CD105, CD166, CD54, CD55, CD13 and CD44, while the markers for hematopoietic stem cells (CD34, CD45, CD14, CD31, and CD133) are negative. According to the properties of cellular surface markers, both magnetic microbead and flow cytometry can be utilized to isolate MSCs, because they are dependent on antigen-antibody reactions. Using these methods, the separated cells are more uniform. Since isolation procedures by flow cytometry cannot be performed under sterile conditions, the magnetic microbead method is adopted to isolate and further culture MSCs. But the cost and technical requirements have limited the wide application of these methods.

1.2 Cell Culture

The culture method is based on the principle of adherent growth by marrow-derived, fibroblast-like cells to the plastic substrate of a culture plate or flask, while marrow-derived hematopoietic cells remain suspended and are discarded during the exchange of the culture medium. Cultured MSCs in the primary culture are heterogeneous and fusiform or fibroblast-like then generally form colonies in the secondary culture. Culture methods for isolated rat MSCs are as follows (the procedures are similar with human MSCs).

1.2.1 Materials

Dubelcco's modified Eagle's medium (DMEM) supplemented with 100 U ml^{-1} penicillin G and 100 U ml^{-1} streptomycin; fetal bovine serum (FBS, Gibco) incubated at 56 ℃ to inactivate compliments (some investigators think heat-inactivation is unnecessary); 0.25% trypsin or supplemented with 0.02% EDTA (ethylene diamine tetra-acetate); sterile phosphate buffered solution (PBS).

1.2.2 Procedures

For the primary culture, the medium should be discarded to remove non-adherent cells after the first 24~48 hours, and every 4~5 days thereafter. Cells will present themselves as fusiform or fibroblast-like on the culture surface after 7 days seeding (Fig. 1.3 A,B). In general it takes 12~14 days for primary cells to form colonies and grow over 80%~90% confluence on the surface of the flask or plate. Once the cells are confluent over 85% of culture surface, they are passaged into a new flask or onto a new plate. The old culture medium containing cellular metabolism products should be discarded, and sterile PBS applied to wash away the residue. Cells are trypsinized with 0.25% trypsin (or supplemented with 0.02% EDTA) for 3~5 minutes at 37 ℃, terminating with DMEM (with 10% FBS) and harvested after centrifugation. PBS washing may be repeated two to three times and the cells collected between each washing step by centrifugation at 400 g for 10 minutes. Cells are resuspended by DMEM supplemented with 10% FBS, counted and plated at a density of $(5\sim7)\times10^5$ ml^{-1} (or one to 2~3 new flasks). The intervals for exchange of the culture medium and passage are associated with the growth rate of cultured cells. During the exchange of the old medium, 3~10 times passaged cells, specifically MSCs, are deprived of non-adherent cells. MSCs *ex vivo* can be identified as fusiform or fibroblast-like, growing adherently on the surface of the culture. The cell has 2∼3 big nuclei that are flat or round and may slightly protrude into the cytoplasm (Fig. 1.3 C). After 10∼12 days in culture, the cells grow confluently on the surface of the flask or plate and form intercellular fusion, often in radiate or swirl patterns that may be confused with non-MSCs.

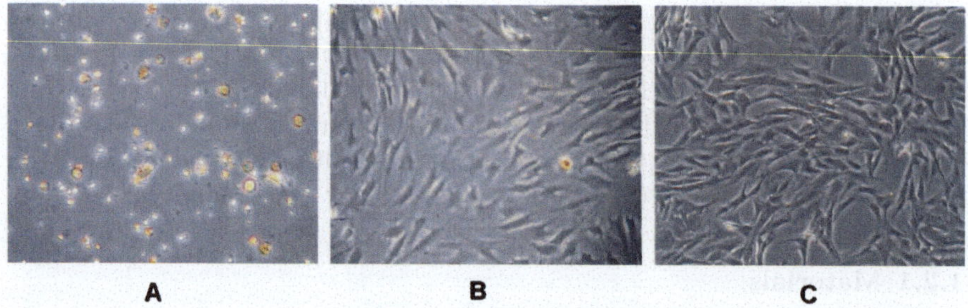

Fig. 1.3. Morphology of rat MSCs in culture system. Under contrast phase microscope, the representative morphology of MSCs isolated from bone marrow and cultured *ex vivo* at Day 1 and Day 7 is shown in Fig. 1.3 A and B, C presents MSCs at Passage 3.

1.3 Cell Cryopreservation and Thawing

As with other cell lines, MSCs can be cryopreserved and thawed. Cryopreservation and thawing may slightly injure MSCs, but has no significant effect on the viability, multipotent differentiation or biological characteristics of these cells. The viability of cryopreserved MSCs is approximately 90%.

Direct cryopreservation without any reagents, will cause intra and extracellular H_2O to form ice crystals, which are harmful to MSCs. Like other damage, such as mechanical injury, electrolyte disturbance, dehydration, pH changes, and protein denaturation, crystalization may lead to cell death. Protective reagents in the medium can lower the freezing point and let intracellular H_2O out of the cells before being frozen. Also, keeping cryopreserved cells at less than –130 ℃ can inhibit the formation of ice crystals. Thawing rapidly through the damage point (approximately –5∼0 ℃) allows for normal cell growth and viability. Cryopreservation reagents, including dimethylsulfoxide (DMSO) and glycerol, should dissolve easily, have a low molecular weight, good intracellular penetration and no cytotoxicity. The choice of cryoprotective agents depends on the type of cells. For most cells, glycerol is a nice choice that has less cytotoxicity than DMSO, while the latter has better intracellular penetration and is more suitable for larger cells, particularly from protists.

1.3.1 Materials

Dubelcco's modified Eagle's medium (DMEM) supplemented with 100 U ml^{-1} penicillin G and 100 U ml^{-1} streptomycin; fetal bovine serum (FBS, Gibco) incubated at 56 °C to inactivate compliments; 0.25% trypsin or supplemented with 0.02% EDTA; sterile phosphate buffered solution (PBS); cryopreservation solution (DMEM supplemented with 10% DMSO and 10% FBS); centrifuge tubes, cryovials, parafilm, etc.

1.3.2 Procedures

For the freezing process, MSCs at Passage 2∼3 are healthy (<90% viability), eugenic, and suitable for cytopreservation. The culture medium should be changed one day before cryopreservation. Cells are detached from the substrate of the flasks by 0.25% trypsin supplemented with 0.02% EDTA, and harvested after centrifugation at 1,000 rpm for 5 minutes at room temperature. Cells are resuspended in prepared cryopreservation solution at a density of 1×10^6 ml^{-1} and divided into cryovials at 1 ml/vial. Cryovials are then parafilmed and labelled with the cell type, date and operator. Once in the cryovials, MSCs are subjected to a sequential cooling process. Cryovials should be cooled at 4 °C for 10 minutes, –20 °C for 30 minutes, –80 °C for 2∼3 days, and then stored in liquid nitrogen.

The procedure for thawing cryopreserved cells begins with the cryovials being removed from liquid nitrogen and rapidly stirred in a 37 °C water bath, taking care not to infuse samples with water. Melted cells are transferred to centrifuge tubes filled with DMEM (10% FBS), and centrifuged at 1,000 rpm for 10 minutes at room temperature. Centrifugation at a lower speed can prevent mechanical injury. The supernatant is discarded and cells are harvested and resuspended in the growth medium. Once transferred to the plates or flasks at a density of 2×10^6 ml^{-1}, cells are incubated at 37 °C with 5% CO_2. The culture medium should be changed in 24 hours. Most cells will grow adherently within 24 hours and present fibroblast or fusiform, with no significant difference in proliferation or morphology.

References

Abildgaard U (1966) Acceleration of fibrin polymerization by dextran and ficoll. Interaction with calcium and plasma proteins. Scand J Clin Lab Invest, 18(5):518-524

Becker AJ, McCulloch EA, Till JE (1963) Cytological demonstration of the clonal nature of spleen colonies derived from transplanted mouse marrow cells. Nature, 197: 452-454

Bernardo ME, Emons JA, Karperien M, Nauta AJ, Willemze R, Roelofs H, Romeo S, Marchini A, Rappold GA, Vukicevic S, Locatelli F, Fibbe WE (2007) Human mesenchymal stem cells derived from bone marrow display a better chondrogenic differentiation compared with other sources. Connect Tissue Res, 48(3):132-140

Campagnoli C, Roberts IA, Kumar S, Bennett PR, Bellantuono I, Fisk NM (2001) Identification of mesenchymal stem/progenitor cells in human first-trimester fetal blood, liver and bone marrow. Blood, 98(8):2396-2402

Erices A, Conget P, Minguell JJ (2000) Mesenchymal progenitor cells in human umbilical cord blood. Br J Haematol, 109(1):235-242

Friedenstein AJ, Piatetzky S II, Petrakova KV (1966) Osteogenesis in transplants of bone marrow cells. J Embryol Exp Morphol, 16(3):381-390

Friedenstein AJ, Deriglasova UF, Kulagina NN, Panasuk AF, Rudakowa SF, Luria EA, Ruadkow IA (1974) Precursors for fibroblasts in different populations of hematopoietic cells as detected by the *in vitro* colony assay method. Exp Hematol, 2(2): 83-92

Friedman MS, Long MW, Hankenson KD (2006) Osteogenic differentiation of human mesenchymal stem cells is regulated by bone morphogenetic protein-6. J Cell Biochem, 98(3):538-554

Gerson SL (1999) Mesenchymal stem cells: no longer second class marrow citizens. Nat Med, 5(3):262-264

Huang ZY, Ge JB, Yang S, Zhang SH, Huang RC, Jin H, Zeng MS, Sun AJ, Qian JY, Zou YZ (2007) *In vivo* cardiac magntic resonance imaging of superparamagnetic iron oxides-labeled mesenchymal stem cells in swines. Zhonghua Xin Xue Guan Bing Za Zhi, 35(4): 344-349

Laurent TC, Pertoft H (1980) Physical chemical characterization of Percoll. III. Sodium binding. J. Colloidal Interface Sci, 76:142-145

Laurent TC, Pertoft H, Nordli O (1980a) Physical chemical characterization of Percoll. I. Particle weight of the colloid. J. Colloid Interface Sci, 76:124-132

Laurent TC, Ogston AJG, Pertoft H, Carlsson B (1980b) Physical chemical characterization of Percoll. II. Size and interaction of colloidal particles. J Colloid Interface Sci, 76:133-141

Lee OK, Kuo TK, Chen WM, Lee KD, Hsieh SL, Chen TH (2004) Isolation of multipotent mesenchymal stem cells from umbilical cord blood. Blood, 103(5):1669-1675

Majumdar MK, Thiede MA, Mosca JD, Moorman M, Gerson SL (1998) Phenotypic and functional comparison of cultures of marrow-derived mesenchymal stem cells (MSCs) and stromal cells. J Cell Physiol, 176(1):57-66

Niu LL, Zheng M, Cao F, Xie C, Li HM, Yue W, Gao YH, Bai CX, Zhu SJ, Pei XT (2004) Migration and differentiation of exogenous rat mesenchymal stem cells engrafted into normal and injured hearts of rats. Zhonghua Yi Xue Za Zhi, 84(1):38-42

Pittenger MF, Mackay AM, Beck SC, Jaiswal RK, Douglas R, Mosca JD, Moorman MA, Simonetti DW, Craig S, Marshak DR (1999) Multilineage potential of adult human mesenchymal stem cells. Science, 284(5411):143-147

Prockop DJ (1997) Marrow stromal cells as stem cells for nonhematopoietic tissues. Science, 276(5309):71-74

Sanchez-Ramos J, Song S, Cardozo-Pelaez F, Hazzi C, Stedeford T, Willing A, Freeman TB, Saporta S, Janssen W, Patel N, Cooper DR, Sanberg PR (2000) Adult bone marrow stromal cells differentiate into neural cells *in vitro*. Exp Neurol, 164(2):247-256

Sila-Asna M, Bunyaratvej A, Maeda S, Kitaguchi H, Bunyaratavej N (2007) Osteoblast differentiation and bone formation gene expression in strontium-inducing bone marrow mesenchymal stem cell. Kobe J Med Sci, 53(1-2):25-35

Siminovitch L, McCulloch EA, Till JE (1963) The distribution of colony-forming cells among spleen colonies. Journal of Cellular and Comparative Physiology, 62:327-336

Suva D, Garavaglia G, Menetrey J, Chapuis B, Hoffmeyer P, Bernheim L, Kindler V (2004) Non-hematopoietic human bone marrow contains long-lasting, pluripotential mesenchymal stem cells. J Cell Physiol, 198(1):110-118

Toma C, Pittenger MF, Cahill KS, Byrne BJ, Kessler PD (2002) Human mesenchymal stem cells differentiate to a cardiomyocyte phenotype in the adult murine heart. Circulation, 105(1):93-98

Xie XJ, Wang JA, Cao J, Zhang X (2006) Differentiation of bone marrow mesenchymal stem cells induced by myocardial medium under hypoxic conditions. Acta Pharmacol Sin, 27(9):1153-1158

2

MSCs Identification

Xinyang Hu[1]

[1]Sir Run Run Shaw Hospital, Zhejiang University College of Medicine, Hangzhou,China
E-mail: hxy0507@hotmail.com

Abstract: Human bone marrow MSCs represents a phenotypically homogeneous cell population that share an identical phenotype with marrow adventitial reticular cells. When an extensive panel of markers is used to characterize MSCs, it appears that the diverse MSC markers described in different laboratories are expressed on the same cell population. Although investigators speak of a number of specific MSC markers, a true marker of MSC "stemness" and multipotentiality has not yet been defined since culture-expanded MSCs may lose some of these markers, but remain multipotential. This chapter will introduce the criteria and some comments on human MSCs defined by International Society for Cellular Therapy (ISCT).

Mesenchymal stem cells (MSCs) are multipotent progenitor cells (Horwitz et al, 2005). During the last two decades, although increasing interest has occurred in the research field of MSCs, different researchers have considered the defining characteristics of MSCs differently. The different methods of MSCs isolation and expansion make it difficult to compare the results of these studies.

2.1 Minimal Criteria

To address this issue, the Mesenchymal and Tissue Stem Cell Committee of the International Society for Cellular Therapy (ISCT) proposes a set of standards to define human MSCs (Dominci et al, 2006). Three criteria are involved to define MSCs as follows.

- Adherent growth to plastic plate or flask
  MSCs must be plastic-adherent when cultured under the standard conditions.
- Specific surface antigen expression
  Surface antigen expression allows for a rapid identification of a cell population. More than 95% of the MSCs must express CD105, CD73 and CD90, as assessed by flow cytometry. To assure that MSCs are not confounded by other types of cells, especially hematopoietic progenitor cells, these cells must also show the absence of some antigen expressions, such as CD45, CD34, CD14 (or $CD11_b$), CD79 (or CD19) and human leucocyte antigen (HLA) Class II (less than 2% should express).
- Multipotent differentiation
  The capacity of tri-lineage differentiation is the most unique biological property for MSCs identification. These cells must be able to differentiate into osteoblasts, adipocytes and chondroblasts under standard differentiating culture conditions *in vitro*.

2.2 Some Comments of the Criteria

- The above criteria only apply to human MSCs identification. MSCs from other species also show plastic-adherence and tri-lineage differentiation, but surface antigen expression is not well characterized and the antigens recommended may not apply to non-human systems.
- As many surface antigen expressions as possible should be tested as deemed importance, including positive and negative markers. The optimum flow cytometric assay should utilize multicolor analyses (i.e. double staining, triple staining, etc.) to demonstrate that individual cells coexpress MSCs markers and lack hematopoietic antigens.
- MSCs express HLA-DR surface molecules in the presence of IFN-γ but not in an unstimulated state. If HLA-DR expression is found, the cells may still be termed MSCs, assuming the other criteria are met, but should be qualified with adjectives, such as "stimulated MSCs"? or other nomenclature to indicate that the cells are not in a baseline state.
- More than 95% positive expression of CD105, CD73, CD90 and less than 2% expression of hematopoietic antigens should be considered as minimal guidelines. A greater level of cell purity may be required for some special experiments. Novel surface markers could lead to modifications of these criteria.

2.3 Other Methods

2.3.1 Morphology Characteristics

Cultured MSCs exhibit spindle or triangular-shaped cell bodies that differ from round hematopoietic cells (Mets and Verdonk, 1981) (Fig. 2.1). It is reported that primary human MSCs isolated by immunomagnetic selection consist of three main phenotypes: 10%~20% of the population are large flat cells (20~50 μm), approximately 80% are small elongated cells (around 7 μm), and 5%~10% are small round cells which can be observed up to Passage 2, at which point they transform into the 7 μm fraction (Lagar'kova et al, 2006).

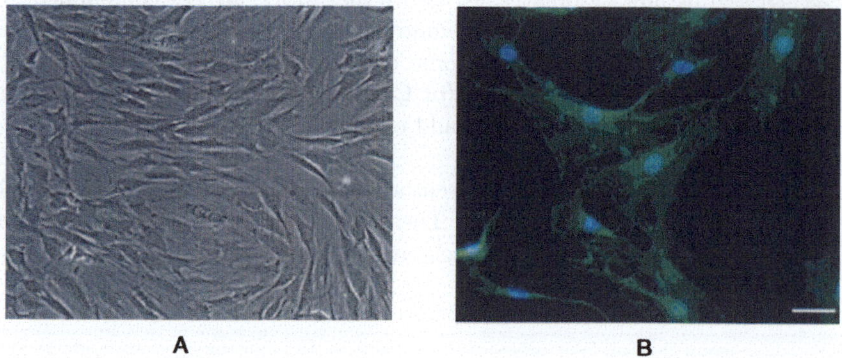

Fig. 2.1. Figure A represents bone marrow MSCs from a rat, while figure B represents bone marrow MSCs from a GFP reporter transgenic mouse

2.3.2 Other Markers

2.3.2.1 SB-10

The specific SB-10 antigen is identified as CD166 (activated leukocyte-cell adhesion molecular, ALCAM), which plays an important role in the progression of osteogenic differentiation (Bruder et al, 1997). Once MSCs differentiate to osteoblasts and express cell surface alkaline phosphotase, SB-10 antigen disappears (Bruder et al, 1998).

2.3.2.2 SH-2, SH-3, SH-4

The SH-2 is an epitope present in CD105 (Barry et al, 1999), while the SH-3 and SH-4 epitopes are present in CD73 (Barry et al, 2001). These antigens disappear upon osteogenic or stromagenic differentiation, and aren't expressed in hematopoietic cells (Haynesworth et al, 1992). Initial studies suggested that these antibodies might be used as reagents for the selection and screening of MSCs populations isolated from bone marrow. However, these antigens are also expressed in other cells.

2.3.2.3 Neural Ganglioside GD2

Recently, Caridad Martinez and colleagues have demonstrated by immunocytochemistry and flow cytometry that neural ganglioside GD2 is expressed on both expanded MSCs in the cultured system and newly isolated MSCs from bone marrow, as well as adipose tissue (Martinez et al, 2007). RT-PCR analysis showed expression of mRNA for GD2 synthase, an essential enzyme for GD2 biosynthesis, which further supported the finding that GD2 is expressed in MSCs. Of note, MSCs are the only cells within normal marrow that express GD2. Thereby, GD2 appears to be the first reported single surface marker that uniquely distinguishes MSCs from other marrow elements (Martinez et al, 2007).

2.3.2.4 SSEA-4

SSEA-4, a stage-specific embryonic antigen previously thought to mark specifically human embryonic stem cells and very early cleavage to blastocyst stage embryos, also identifies an adult mesenchymal stem cell population. Eun J. Gang reported that with the elimination of hematopoietic cells in the culture, SSEA-4 expression gradually increased. Standardized preparations of MSCs obtained from the Tulane Center for Gene Therapy have high levels of SSEA-4 expression. Flow cytometric analysis showed that hematopoietic cells were absent in SSEA-4^+ sorted cells. So SSEA-4 can be used for the prospective isolation of MSCs from the whole bone marrow aspirates (Gang et al, 2007).

2.4 Conclusion

In conclusion, there is no single method or surface marker to identify MSCs thus far. We should apply the minimal criteria for defining multi-potent mesenchymal stem cells as reported by the International Society for Cellular Therapy (ISCT), which combines morphology, surface markers and multiple differentiation potentials to identify MSCs.

References

Barry FP, Boynton RE, Haynesworth S, Murphy JM, Zaia J (1999) The monoclonal antibody SH-2, raised against human mesenchymal stem cells, recognizes an epitope on endoglin (CD105). Biochem Biophys Res Commun, 265(1):134-139

Barry F, Boynton R, Murphy M, Haynesworth S, Zaia J (2001) The SH-3 and SH-4 antibodies recognize distinct epitopes on CD73 from human mesenchymal stem cells. Biochem Biophys Res Commun, 289(2):519-524

Bruder SP, Horowitz MC, Mosca JD, Haynesworth SE (1997) Monoclonal antibodies reactive with human osteogenic cell surface antigens. Bone, 21(3):225-235

Bruder SP, Kraus KH, Goldberg VM, Kadiyala S (1998) The effect of implants loaded with autologous mesenchymal stem cells on the healing of canine segmental bone defects. J Bone Joint Surg Am, 80(7):985-996

Dominici M, Le Blanc K, Mueller I, Slaper-Cortenbach I, Marini F, Krause D, Deans R, Keating A, Prockop Dj, Horwitz E (2006) Minimal criteria for defining multipotent mesenchymal stromal cells. The International Society for Cellular Therapy position statement. Cytotherapy, 8(4):315-317

Gang EJ, Bosnakovski D, Figueiredo CA, Visser JW, Perlingeiro RC (2007) SSEA-4 identifies mesenchymal stem cells from bone marrow. Blood, 109(4): 1743-1751

Haynesworth, SE, Baber MA, Caplan AI (1992) Cell surface antigens on human marrow-derived mesenchymal cells are detected by monoclonal antibodies. Bone, 13(1):69-80

Horwitz EM, Le Blanc K, Dominici M, Mueller I, Slaper-Cortenbach I, Marini FC, Deans RJ, Krause DS, Keating A (2005) Clarification of the nomenclature for MSC. The International Society for Cellular Therapy position statement. Cytotherapy, 7(5):393-395

Lagar'kova MA, Lyakisheva AV, Filonenko ES, Volchkov PY, Rubtsova KV, Gerasimov YV, Chailakhyan RK, Kiselev SL (2006) Characteristics of human bone marrow mesenchymal stem cells isolated by immunomagnetic selection. Bull Exp Biol Med, 141(1):112-116

Martinez C, Hofmann TJ, Marino R, Dominici M, Horwitz EM (2007) Human bone marrow mesenchymal stromal cells express the neural ganglioside GD2: a novel surface marker for the identification of MSCs. Blood, 109(10):4245-4248

Mets T, Verdonk G (1981) *In vitro* aging of human bone marrow derived stromal cells. Mech Ageing Dev, 16(1):81-89

3

Biological Characteristics of MSCs

Aina He[1], Shaoping Wang[2], Tielong Chen[3], Jiahui Li[4], Xianbao Liu[5]

[1,2,5]Second Affiliated Hospital, Zhejiang University College of Medicine, Hangzhou, China
E-mail: [1]happybabyfp@hotmail.com
[2]wang_shaoping@hotmail.com
[5]liuxb2009@hotmail.com
[3]Hangzhou Hospital of Tranditional Chinese Medicine, Hangzhou, China
E-mail: ctlppp@sohu.com
[4]Chinese-Japan Friendship Hospital, Beijing, China
E-mail: veighlee@hotmail.com

Abstract: Recent advancements in tissue engineering and regenerative medicine have highlighted MSCs as a potential source of cells which would differentiate to a variety of tissue tailored to individual needs. This chapter briefly outlines the current status of MSCs, focusing on their biological characteristics and potential for clinical applications.

3.1 Surface Markers and Paracrine Characteristics

3.1.1 Surface Markers

MSCs have been defined by their plastic-adherent growth and subsequent expansion under specific culture conditions, by a panel of nonspecific surface antigens and by their *in vitro* and *in vivo* differentiation potential. MSC transdifferentiation into myocytes, osteoblasts, adipocytes and chondrocytes by different inducers have been widely demonstrated. In contrast, human fibroblasts cannot transdifferentiate into other lineage cells, except fibrocytes. A CD (cluster of differentiation) molecule is a kind of membrane antigen associated with cell development, differentiation and activation. MSCs have been identified as expressing CD29, CD44, CD90, CD105, and lacking hematopoietic lineage markers and HLA-DR (Dominici et al, 2006). In general, MSC refers to bone marrow-derived cells, while similar populations can also be obtained from other tissues, such as adipose umbilical cord blood and peripheral blood, connective tissues of the dermis, and skeletal muscle. The biological characteristics of MSCs derived from other tissues are not the same as those from bone marrow. Hereby we discuss the surface markers of bone marrow-derived MSCs.

Multiple studies have focused on the identification of specific surface markers on MSCs, in an effort to effectively isolate MSCs. For instance, a high expression of CD105, CD73, and CD90 is used as one of minimal criteria to identify human MSCs. Scores of monoclonal antibodies have been raised in an effort to provide reagents for the characterization and isolation of human MSCs. It has been demonstrated that at least three types of surface markers are expressed on MSCs (Jootar et al, 2006) (Table 3.1), including adhesion molecules, extra-cellular matrix proteins, cytokine and growth factor receptors. In addition, a series of antibody binding sites exists on the membrane of human MSCs, including prolyl-4-hydroxylase, vimentin, desmin, nestin, CD13, collagen IV, osteopontin, osteonectin, bone sialoprotein II and endogenous alkaline phosphatase to name a few. The expression of these cell markers depends not only on species, original tissues and individuals MSCs, but also on the different status of the cell cycle. For rat MSCs, there is high expression of CD44, CD90, c-kit and stemcell antigen-1 (sca-1) (Xie et al, 2006; Uemura et al, 2006) and low expression of CD34, VE-cadherin, Flk-1 and c-met (Uemura et al, 2006). MSCs in different generations may present different antigen, i.e., nestin as an immature marker will be gradually absent during subsequent passages.

Surface markers of MSCs can be changed after transdifferentiation. For example, rat MSCs, after specific induction, can differentiate into cells with the Schwann cell (SC) phenotypes according to their morphology and immunoreactivities to SC surface markers including S-100, glial fibrillary acidic protein (GFAP) and low-affinity nerve growth factor receptor (p75). The expression of surface markers can also decrease or increase during the differentiation, and

Table 3.1. Surface markers of human bone marrow MSCs

Surface Markers	CD Molecules	Biological Properties	Ref.
Cytokine and Growth Factor Receptors			
Interleukin(IL) receptors IL-1R,IL-3R,IL-4R,IL-6R,IL-7R	CD121, CD123, CD124, CD126, CD127	Differentiation Immune Regulation	(Erices et al, 2002; Silva et al, 2003)
stem cell factor receptor(SCFR)	CD117	Differentiation	(Gagari et al, 2006)
leukemia inhibitor factor receptor(LIFR)		Differentiation	(Falconi et al, 2007)
INF-interferon receptor	CDw119	Immune Regulation	(Krampera et al, 2003)
Tumor necrosis factor receptor: TNF-α_1R, -α_2R	CD120a,b	Anti-inflammation	(Ortiz et al, 2007)
Transforming growth factor:TGF-β_1R,-β_2R		Activation Adhesion	(Moon et al, 2007)
Fibroblast growth factor receptor(FGFR)		Differentiation	(Chiou et al, 2006)
Platelet-derived growth factor receptor, (PDGFR)	CD140a	Migration Angiogenesis	(Ball et al, 2007)
Epidermal growth factor receptor(EGFR)		Proliferation	(Krampera et al, 2005)
Adhesion Molecules			
Intercellular adhesion molecule: ICAM-1,2,3	CD54, CD102, CD50	Proliferation	(Honczarenko et al, 2006)
Activated leukocyte cell adhesion molecule (ALCAM)		Differentiation	(Risbud et al, 2004)
Vascular cell adhesion molecule (VCAM)	CD106	Differentiation	(Gang et al, 2006)
Endoglin	CD105	Differentiation	(Barry et al, 1999)
Hyaluronate receptor	CD44	Migration	(Zhu et al, 2006)
Extracellular Matrix (ECM)			
Fibronectin		Differentiation	(Djouad et al, 2007)
Laminin			(Silva et al, 2003)
Hyaluronan		Migration	(Lisignoli et al, 2006)
Integrins		Migration	(Ip et al, 2007)
Other Markers			
src homology protein: SH-2,3,4	CD105, CD73, CD73		(Peiffer et al, 2007)
Stromal-derived factor-1(STRO-1)		Differentiation	(Caddick et al, 2006)
Thymus cell antigen-1(Thy-1)		Differentiation	(Caddick et al, 2006)
P75			
SSEA-3, SSEA-4			(Jones et al, 2004)
D7			

some surface markers indicate a differentiation potential, as integrin subunits α_{10}, a potential marker to predict the chondrogenic differentiation state of MSCs.

3.1.2 Paracrine Characteristics of MSCs

As one of many multi-potent adult stem cells, the potential plasticity and self-renewal characteristics of MSCs make them a possible candidate for clinical tissue regeneration. Most of the study results consistently demonstrate that MSCs transplantation can improve cardiac function and retard ventricular remodeling in myocardial infarcted (MI) animals (Orlic et al, 2001b; Wang et al, 2004; Wang et al, 2006a). Many clinical trials have also demonstrated that the MSCs therapy is helpful for patients who have suffered an MI or heart failure (Schächinger et al, 2006; Aussmus et al, 2002; Wang et al, 2005; Wang et al, 2006b). The mechanisms behind these therapeutic effects have not been clearly defined. There exists an intense debate over differentiation versus cell fusion, which is much more complex than previously anticipated.

Recently, the paracrine effect of MSCs transplantation has been emphasized. An array of cytokines and growth factors are involved in paracrine effects of MSCs therapy. These factors are helpful in protecting cardiomyocytes from apoptosis and necrosis, promoting angiogenesis in infarcted myocardium, retarding matrix remodeling and augmenting circulating MSCs recruitment (as shown in Table 3.2). Transplanted MSCs can upregulate multiple growth factors in the cardiac microenvironment, such as the vascular endothelial growth factor (VEGF, which promotes angiogenesis, increases blood flow, and decreases apoptosis), the fibroblast growth factor (FGF, which acts as an angiogenic, antifibrotic and antiapoptotic factor), the hepatocyte growth factor (HGF, which has angiogenic, antiapoptotic, mitogenic and antifibrotic effects), adrenomedullin (which also has angiogenic, antiapoptotic and antifibrotic effects), and the insulin-like growth factor-1 (IGF-1, which promotes cardiomyogenesis, antiapoptosis, positive inotropic effects) (Uemura et al, 2006; Wang et al, 2004; Gnecchi et al, 2006; Li et al, 2002).

However, the paracrine effects of MSCs are still being challenged. If paracrine factors are the key agents, could isolating and delivering such factors in high concentrations result in stable or increased protection? The following issues should be considered: (1)The secreted components and their proportions are still unknown, so the ideal “cocktail” is difficult to anticipate. (2)Would MSCs secrete cytokines into ischemic myocardium stably, directly and consistently? (3)The regeneration properties of MSCs are still being considered. (4)Could the secreted cytokines play a role in MSCs (an autocrine effect)? According to the above issues, we propose that modifications of MSCs in order to enhance the survival of engrafted MSCs and secrete more paracrine factors might result in increased cardioprotection.

Table 3.2. Cytokines secreted by human or rat bone marrow-derived MSCs

Human MSCs	Rat MSCs
Interleukin:IL-6,-7,-8,-11,-12,-14,-15	Vascular endothelial growth factor (VEGF)
Stem cell factor (SCF)	Hepatocyte growth factor (HGF)
Leukemia inhibitory Factor (LIF)	Insulin-like growth factor-1(IGF-1)
Stromal-derived factor: SDF-1	Adrenomedlin
FMS-like tyrosine kinase 3: Flt-3 Ligand	SDF
Macrophage colony-stimulating factor (MCSF)	Fibroblast growth factor (bFGF)
Transforming growth factor β (TGF-β)	Matrix metalloproteinases (MMP)
Bone morphogeneic protein 4 (BMP-4)	Angiopoetin
oncostatin M (OSM)	TGF-β
	Platelet-derived growth factor (PDGF)

3.2 Electrophysiological Properties of MSCs and Their Electric Coupling with Cardiomyocytes

Ion channels are membrane proteins, found in both excitable and nonexcitable cells, which control the basic activity of bioelectricity. More than 340 human genes are thought to encode proteins of ion channels, which play important roles in such diverse processes as nerve and muscle excitation, hormone secretion, cell proliferation, sensory transduction, learning and memory, regulation of blood pressure, salt and water balance, cell migration, fertilization and cell death. Consequently, functional defects of ion channels often have profound physiological effects. With the development of biophysical and molecular biology, especially the marriage of the patch clamp technique and molecular cloning with gene mutation and expression, studies of ion channels have been pushed rapidly promoted in life science.

MSCs, as nonexcitable cells, can express various types of ion channels. Under given conditions, they can transdifferentiate into excitable-like cells such as cardiac myocytes. Cell proliferation and survival, with an appropriate function in ischemic tissues, as well as interaction with adjacent cardiac myocytes, is crucial in cell regeneration therapy. This review introduces ion channels in MSCs and the electrical coupling between MSCs and host cardiomyocytes.

3.2.1 Characterization of Ion Channels in MSCs

The expression of ion channels is variform in MSCs. A distinct single cell may express one or various types of ion channels. Some MSCs express ion channels within the physiological range of potentials, while some do not. Gene expression is not always consistent with the functional expression of ion current. Different genes have distinct phenotypes of ion channels. Bone marrow-derived MSCs from different species also present different ion channels.

3.2.1.1 Potassium Channels (K^+ Channels)

K^+ channels are a most diverse class of ion channels in the cytoplasmic membrane. To date, no less than 20 distinct K^+ channel currents have been identified in primary tissues. The functional and structural diversity of K^+ channels has been further elucidated by molecular cloning technique. K^+ channels are found to be abundant in undifferentiated MSCs.

Two groups have depicted the electrophysiological properties of human MSCs (Heubach et al, 2003; Li et al, 2005). Two types of K^+ currents, i.e. Ca^{2+} activated K^+ currents (IK_{Ca}) and delayed rectifier K^+ currents (IK_{DR}), can be recorded in most human MSCs, and often coexist with other ionic currents in a single cell (Fig. 3.1).

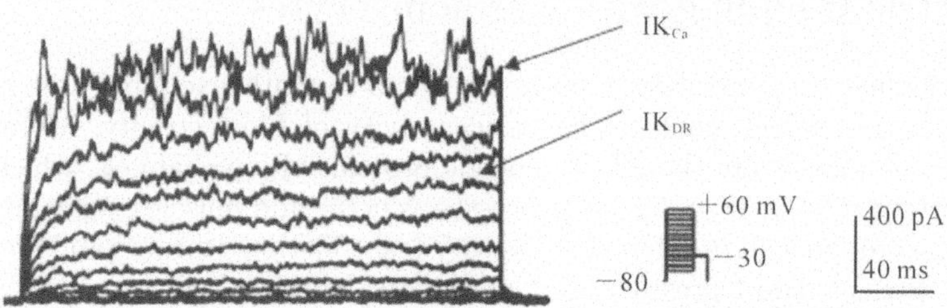

Fig. 3.1. Membrane currents were recorded in a representative human MSCs. It shows two components of outward currents are present: one is a slowly activating current like delayed rectifier K^+ currents (IK_{DR}) at potentials from –30 mV to +30 mV, and the other is a rapid activating current with noisy oscillation like Ca^{2+} activated K^+ currents (IK_{Ca}) at potentials from +40 mV to +60 mV.

IK_{Ca} has the characteristics of: (1) a rapid activation at potentials of more than +40 mV, voltage-dependent currents with noisy oscillation; (2) sensitivity to the specific large-conductance Ca^{2+}-activated channel blocker iberiotoxin; (3) a high expression level of MaxiK mRNA.

IK_{DR} has been significantly recorded using high ethylene glycol bis (2-aminoethyl ether) tetraacetic acid (EGTA, 5 mM) in pipette solution and Cd^{2+} in superfusion solution to inhibit the activation of IK_{Ca}. Resting membrane potential is relatively negative (–25~–42 mV) in cells with significant IK_{DR}. IK_{DR} (as shown in Fig. 3.1) is slowly activated with depolarization voltage steps and shows non-inactivation. More negative conditioning potentials and a higher concentration of extracellular Mg^{2+} could slow the activation of IK_{DR}. A non-specific IK blocker, tetraethylammonium (TEA), could significantly inhibit the current with an IC_{50} around 2.0 mM. According to electrophysiological properties such as activated potential, IK_{DR} consists of rapidly activating outward potassium current (IK_r) and slow activating outward potassium current (IK_s), one or both of which can be expressed in cells. Single IK_s expression is more common in cells. IK_{DR} is complemented by the heag1 K^+ channels for the high expression levels of *heag1* mRNA.

In addition, a transient outward K^+ current (Ito) has been recorded in a small fraction of cells (about 8%). Other types of K^+ currents, including hyperpolarization-activated inward current (If), inward rectifier K^+ currents (IK_{ir}), ATP-sensitive K^+ currents (IK_{ATP}), and cardiac acetylcholine-stimulated inward rectifier currents (IK_{Ach}) have not been recorded by patch clamp technique, though the associated mRNA has been detected.

The outward currents recorded in human MSCs could not be blocked by DIDS, a blocker of Cl^- currents, which indicates that no components of Cl^- currents are combined with outward K^+ currents.

3.2.1.2 Calcium Channels (Ca^{2+} Channels)

It has been demonstrated that Ca^{2+} plays a crucial role in cell functional regulation, including differentiation and proliferation. Two predominant sources of Ca^{2+} are involved in cell signaling. One is extracellular Ca^{2+} transported across the membrane, the other is Ca^{2+} released from intracelluar storage. Extracellular Ca^{2+} transport across the membrane occurs via two distinct pathways, voltage-operated Ca^{2+} channels (VOCCs), and agonist-dependent Ca^{2+} entry pathways, which are voltage-independent and also called store-operated Ca^{2+} channels (SOCCs).

Many investigators have detected Ca^{2+} currents of L-type VOCCs ($I_{Ca,L}$) in a small population (about 15%) of undifferentiated human MSCs (Fig. 3.2). I-V relationship of $I_{Ca,L}$ displays the current peaked at 0 mV with a density of 0.8±0.3 pA/pF. The currents can be sensitively inhibited by nifedipine. *CACNA1C* mRNA of the L-type Ca^{2+} channel (but not the T-type Ca^{2+} channel *CACNA1G*) has been detected in human MSCs.

SOCCs are the predominant Ca^{2+} pathway from the membrane in most of human MSCs, while VOCCs make little contribution to Ca^{2+} entry (Kawano et al, 2002). The currents of SOCC can be recorded by the whole-cell patch-clamp technique, and activated via an inositol (1, 4, 5)-trisphosphate(InsP3)-related pathway.

Ca^{2+} released from intracellular storage occurs primarily from the endoplasmic reticulum (ER) wherein two functionally distinct Ca^{2+} release channels have been identified, namely InsP3R and RyR. Human MSCs have spontaneous $[Ca^{2+}]$i oscillations without agonists or other stimuli. The intracellular Ca^{2+} storage is the major Ca^{2+} source for these oscillations, and Ca^{2+} influx (mostly via SOCCs) is required to refill intracellular Ca^{2+} storage and maintain these oscillations. InsP3R is the major contributor to Ca^{2+}

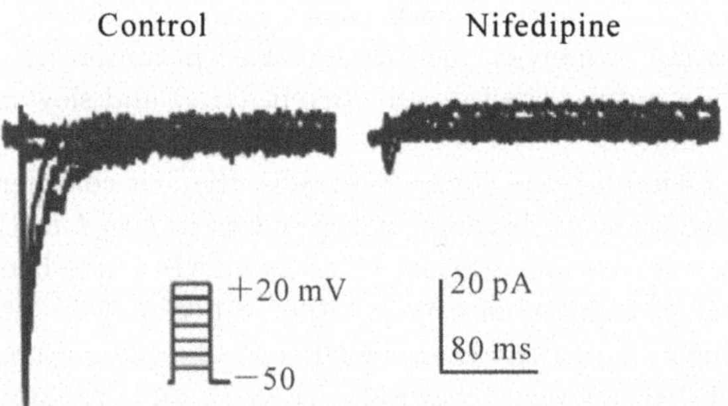

Fig. 3.2. L-type Ca^{2+} current recorded by patch clamp technique under K^+-free conditions in human MSCs. Ca^{2+} currents of L-type VOCCs ($I_{Ca,L}$) activated by 200 ms voltage steps from –40 mV to +10 mV with a holding potential of –50 mV (to inactivate I_{Na}) under control conditions (left panel) and after application of nifedipine for 6 minutes (right panel) in a representative cell.

released from ER, while RyRs molecules are found not to be expressed in undifferentiated MSCs.

3.2.1.3 Sodium Channels (Na^+ Channels)

Voltage-dependent sodium currents (I_{Na}) have been recorded in about 29% of human MSCs, peaked at –15 mV with a threshold potential of –40 mV. The currents are more sensitively blocked by tetrodotoxin (TTX). Multitude mRNA expression of TTX-sensitive Na^+ channel gene *hNE-Na* (but not *SCN5A*) has been detected in human MSCs.

The results of ion channels in undifferentiated human MSCs from different studies are inconsistent. Mareschi and his colleagues (Mareschi et al, 2006) have reported that the only K^+ channel detected in undifferentiated human MSCs is the slow channel activated at extremely unphysiological potentials ($V_{1/2}$ = +168 mV). However, I_{Na} could not been detected in some other experiments.

Different species have distinct phenotypes of these ion channels. In our experiments, most rat MSCs express IK_{DR} (Fig. 3.3) (Wang S et al, 2008; Wang SP et al, 2008). The currents were outward rectifier and voltage-dependent, which could be activated at potentials from positive to –40 mV, rapidly activated and no markedly inactivated. The currents have no detectable tail currents on returning to –80 mV, and could be largely blocked by TEA. IK_{Ca} and I_{to} have also been recorded in a small fraction of rat MSCs. However, no outward currents have been recorded within the physiological potential (from –60 mV to +60 mV) in rat MSCs.

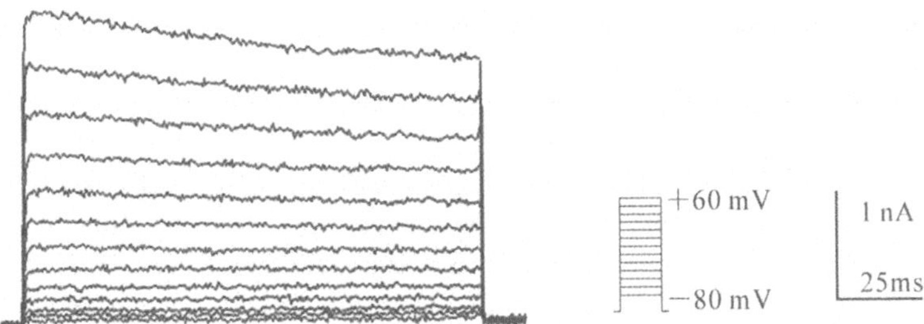

Fig. 3.3. IK_{DR} was recorded in a single rat MSCs by patch clamp technique. The cell was depolarized by a series of test potentials from −60 mV to +60 mV with a holding potential of −80 mV in +10 mV increments.

3.2.2 Why Does an Individual Cell Express Different Currents?

At present, human MSCs are identified by characteristic growth patterns and cell morphology, multipotent differentiation and cell surface markers, such as CD29, CD105 and CD166. However, our studies show a complex distribution of ion channels in human MSCs, making a case for a heterogeneous cell population, although the cells employed were considered relatively homogeneous. Specifically, L-type Ca^{2+} channel, which is critical for excitation-contraction coupling mechanisms in an adult heart, has not been frequently found in human MSCs. The cells might be confounded with a fraction of progenitor cells. Studies of ion channels to reveal functional markers of MSCs might contribute to the further identification of human MSCs and the evaluation of its therapeutic effects both *in vitro* and *in vivo.*

Another possible reason is that ion current expression depends on cell function. For example, activation of K^+ channels hyperpolarizes membrane potential and reduces the cell size. The status of K^+ channels can regulate the cell cycle; by contrast, current expression varies at different phases of the cell cycle.

In addition, slight differences in cell culture conditions, such as antibiotics may influence the different properties of currents.

3.2.3 Electric Coupling of MSCs with Host Cardiomyocytes

Once MSCs are transplanted into the host myocardium, mechanical joints would be present among adjacent host cardiomyocytes (CMCs), adjacent MSCs, and between CMCs and MSCs. Structural and functional integration of injected cells with host myocardium is crucial in achieving a therapeutic effect. Intercellular electrical coupling may influence heart rhythm and thus hemodynamics. Recently, injection of skeletal myoblasts into damaged myocardium in patients suffering from heart failure was found to result in life-threatening ventricular arrhythmias. An absence of electrical coupling via connexin43 between injected skeletal myoblasts and resident CMCs might be the molecular basis of the proarrhythmyogenic effect.

Gap junctions contribute to form intercellular low-resistance pathways allowing for intercellular transport of low molecular traffic (up to 1 kDa) and conduction of electrical impulses, thereby ensuring coordinated propagation of action potentials across the myocardium. Gap junctions consist of connexin40 (Cx40), connexin43 (Cx43), and connexin45 (Cx45), which are localized in the atria, ventricles, and conduction system respectively. Cx43 is the predominant isoform of connexin in gap junctions.

It has been demonstrated that Cx43 is expressed in human MSCs and involved in the formation of functional gap junctions between human MSCs and CMCs, as well as coupled human MSCs. Human MSCs plated into a central acellular channel between two separated cultures of CMCs led to an experimental conduct block. Human MSCs could conduct an electrical signal over a considerable distance for at least 14 days, and thus resynchronize two separated fields of CMCs (Pijnappels et al, 2006). In cardiac tissue, conduction velocity (CV) is determined by cell-to-cell coupling, tissue architecture and excitability. However, the undifferentiated human MSCs are non-excitable cells with rest membrane potential of about –30∼–40 mV. The percentage of human MSCs expression L-type Ca^{2+} channels and sodium channels were rather low, ranging from 15% to 29%. It was found that a TTX-sensitive Na^{+} channel was present, which was associated with *SCN9A* gene expression but not *SCN5A*. Conduction velocity across the human MSCs was about 3.5±0.1 cm/s after 14 days' culture, which was far slower than that across cardiomyocytes (16.8±0.2 cm/s). It is proposed that electrical currents were conducted across human MSCs by electronic conduction via a gap junction without activation of ion channels to maintain electrical propagation across excitable tissues.

Human MSCs have been cocultured with neonatal rat ventricular myocytes (NRVM). More than 10% of MSCs in a co-culture system led to decreased conduction velocity (Chang et al, 2006). Since conduction velocity depends on both gap junction coupling and excitability, it indicates that a decrease in conduction velocity in the co-culture system might be attributed to the inexcitable nature of the MSCs and their ability to act as current sinks. The coupled MSCs with a resting membrane potential of –40 mV could partially depolarize neighboring myocytes, inactivate Na^{+} channels, and decrease conduction velocity.

Furthermore, it was found that reentrant arrhythmias occured in 86% of the co-cluture system with 10% and 20% MSCs. Factors predisposed to reentrant arrhythmias included a heterogeneous distribution of MSCs and electric coupling of inexcitable MSCs with host myocytes. Consequently, MSCs may inactivate Na^{+} channels in myocytes in a heterogeneous fashion. These effects would be aggravated at high pacing rates for incomplete recovery of

Na^+ channels and result in conduction block, wavebreak and reentrant arrhythmias. Reentrant arrhythmias had also been certified *in vivo* by animal models after intramyocardial injection of large numbers of MSCs. MSCs injected into the cardiac microenvironment would delay the activation and recovery process of action potential in the transplanted region. Thereby, high heart rates or premature impulses may encounter refractory tissue in the transplanted area with MSCs, leading to a localized block of impulse propagation and susceptibility to reentry. Reentrant arrhythmias could not be induced in NRVM-only controls or coculture systems containing only 1% human MSCs. In conclusion, the arrhythmogenicity may depend on the number of inexcitable MSCs transplanted into the host myocardium.

Experimental heart failure models were established by injection of adriamycin in rabbits. About 1.0×10^7 of autologous MSCs were introduced into coronary arteries by occluding the root of ascending aorta (Chen et al, 2005). Cell transplantation caused prolongation of activation time (AT) of myocardium and exacerbation of AT dispersion during burst or presystolic pacing, which was more significant in the apex of left ventricle and septum than that in right ventricular outflow tract. It could be partially explained that MSCs were flushed into capillary arteries and migrated into the apex of left ventricle and septum. The electric conduction velocity of myocardium was decreased by the transplanted inexcitable MSCs. One of eight rabbits developed spontaneous ventricular tachycardia and sudden cardiac death.

In cell therapy for myocardial infarction, a sufficient number of MSCs is necessary to improve cardiac function of ischemic myocardium, but more transplanted cells may lead to arrhythmas. In practice, the injected cells tend to resemble the ratio of 1:99 in MSCs/NRVM co-culture system as described above. The safety of MSCs therapy has also been demonstrated in other studies. We have not observed any proarrhythmic effect by intravenous or intracoronary MSCs therapy in animal models or patients with myocardial infarction and dilated cardiomyopathy (Wang et al, 2004, 2005, 2006b; Zhang et al, 2008).

It is indicated by studies from Mills and his colleagues that MSCs transplantation not only does not increase susceptibility to arrhythmias, but also may even exert a protective effect on electrical recovery, not just a mechanical benefit in the setting of myocardial infarction (Mills et al, 2007). In their experiment, 2 millions MSCs infused intravenously were demonstrated to preserve the electrical viability and impulse propagation in the border zone by optical mapping technique in the rat myocardium infarction model.

It has been reported that an arrhythmia inducibility score with MSCs therapy is significantly lower than that for a skeletal myoblast, and tends to be lower than myocardial infarction models without cell therapy (Cohen et al, 2007). One of the reasons is that MSCs, as mentioned previously, can express Cx43 and form functional gap junctions with myocytes. MSCs are expected to effectively interdigitate between islands of surviving myocytes and provide a pathway for current flow (Fig. 3.4). Another possible reason is that MSCs could preserve the injured myocytes both in the border zone and within the infarcted region by several pathways, including decreasing the apoptosis and necrosis of myocytes, promoting proliferation of native myocytes, and transdifferentiating into cardiomyocyte-like cells. Consequently, more native electrical properties are effectively preserved and the similar benefits in mechanical function are achieved.

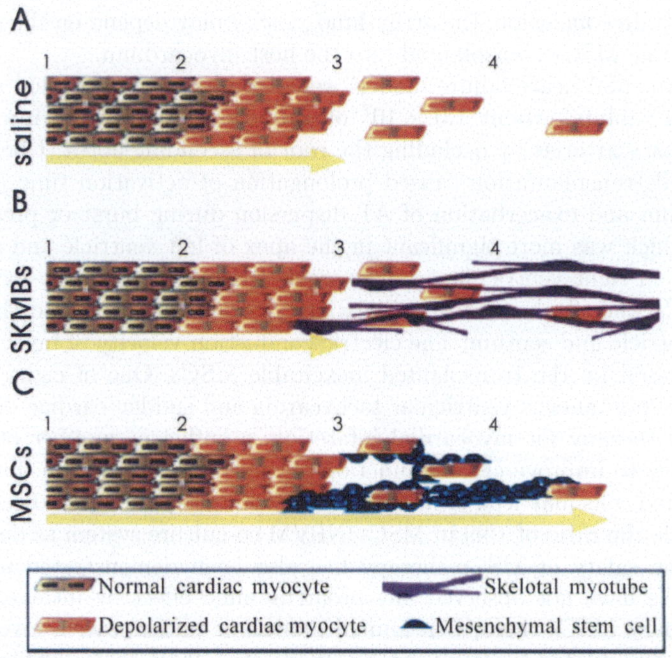

Fig. 3.4. Electrophysiological changes of cellular therapy on infarcted myocardium. (A) After myocardial infarction, cells in the border zone (between 2 and 3) are depolarized, and the few surviving myocytes in the infarcted zone (between 3 and 4) are poorly coupled to the border cells. Electrical current flow to the border region is significantly reduced (arrow in yellow depicts current flow terminating at interface between the border zone and the infarcted zone). (B) When skeletal myoblasts (SKMBs) are transplanted into the infarcted zone, they do not form an electrical couple, and thus do not promote electrical function in the infarcted zone.

(C) Transplanted mesenchymal stem cells (MSCs) couple to the surviving myocytes in the border and infarcted zones, permitting electrical current spread into the latter region (depicted by arrow in yellow which is extending into the infarcted zones). They may also enhance myocardial survival via angiogenesis or promote myocyte proliferation in the infarcted zone by secreting paracrine factors.

Though MSCs exhibit arrhythmogenicity as inexcitable cells when cocultured with excitable cardiomyocytes *in vitro*, they still exert electric benefits after transplantation into infarcted myocardium. The distinct electric properties between cultured cardiomyocytes and surviving myocytes in the border of infarcted zones, when coupled to MSCs, may be responsible. Strategic dispersal of MSCs to the infarcted myocardium may be crucial to achieve electric benefits.

MSCs can express Cx43, the prodominant gap junction protein, and form functional gap junctions between MSCs, as well as between MSCs and myocytes, which are hypothesized to generate pacemaker-like currents to enhance focal ventricular automaticity in animal models. Human MSCs have been transfected with a cardiac pacemaker gene, *mHCN2*, and as a result expressed If-like currents (Potapova et al, 2004). The transfected cells could influence the beating rate *in vitro* when plated onto a coverslip and overlaid with neonatal rat ventricular myocytes. When 10^6 human MSCs transfected with *mHCN2* gene were injected subepicardially into the canine left ventricular wall *in situ* during sinus arrest, 5 out of 6 animals developed spontaneous ventricular rhythms of left-sided origin. Ren and colleagues had explored a new therapy for atrioventricular block (AVB) by MSCs transplantation in canines (Ren et al, 2005). MSCs were differentiated by 5-azacytidine *in vitro*, then were injected in the His bundle area, which had been completely damaged by radiofrequency ablation. After 12 weeks, 2 out of 6 canines with third-degree AVB were alleviated by cell therapy and developed second-degree AVB. Other investigations are focusing on the efficacy of MSCs treatment in symptomatic bradycardia (Tse et al, 2006).

3.3 Proliferation of MSCs and Telomerase Properties

A profound understanding of MSCs biological characteristics has opened the way to their clinical application. The properties of telomeres and telomerase are associated with MSCs proliferation. Telomeres, unique structures at the physical ends of linear eukaryotic chromosomes, were first described by Hermann Muller almost 70 years ago. Telomeres consist of repetitive G-rich sequences and an abundance of associated proteins, which together form a dynamic cap. Telomeres serve multiple functions in preserving chromosome stability; including protecting the ends of chromosome from degradation and preventing chromosomal end fusion. Telomere dysfunction can contribute to chromosomal instability. Telomerase is a specialized RNA-protein complex responsible for the de novo synthesis and maintenance of telomere repeats. It consists of a telomerase RNA component that serves as a template for the addition of repeats, and a protein component (telomerase reverse transcriptase). It has been demonstrated that bone marrow-derived MSCs can transdifferentiate into cells of different organs, such as bone, cartilage, muscle and adipose tissue, exhibiting multi-potent characteristics in some microenvironments. How do telomeres and telomerase affect the biological properties of MSCs? Herein we will introduce them briefly.

3.3.1 Structure and Function of Telomeres and Telomerase

Telomeres are composed of specialized DNA sequences and telomere-binding proteins, located at the ends of linear chromosomes. In humans and other vertebrates, the DNA component of telomeres consists of tandem arrays of the short, repetitive G-rich sequence TTAGGG. Interestingly, telomere lengths differ greatly, even among mammals. For example, human telomeres are 5 to 15 kbp long while those of inbred mice may exceed 60 kbp. Telomeric DNA tracts are dynamic entities which are subject to shorten during cell division. Conversely, telomeres may be elongated through activation of the ribonucleoprotein enzyme telomerase or genetic recombination (Meeker et al, 2004). Several specific proteins are associated to telomeric DNA, including telomerase and the telomeric repeat binding factors 1 and 2 (TRF1, TRF2) which directly bind to the TTAGGG repeat and interact with other factors forming large protein complexes that regulate telomere length and structure. The telomeric repeats contribute to the maintenance of chromosomal integrity and provide a buffer of potentially expendable DNA. The ends of telomeres are protected by telomere-binding proteins, which form a special T-loop (Shay and Wright, 2005). The T-loop can mask telomeres from being recognized as damaged DNA, thereby protecting chromosomal ends from recombination and degradation (Shay and Wright, 2005). In addition, telomeres play an important role in cell apoptosis and proliferation.

Telomerase is a specialized RNA ribonucleoprotein complex, which consists of a telomerase RNA component (TERC) that serves as a template for the synthesis of new telomeric DNA repeats, and a protein component, telomerase reverse transcriptase (TERT). TERT is a type of reverse transcriptase able to synthesize TTAGGG repeats from the RNA template. TERT is highly expressed in all tissues regardless of telomerase activity (Cong, 2002), with cancer cells generally having five-fold higher expressions than normal cells. In the absence of telomerase, chromosomes shorten slightly with every cell division. To maintain cell division continuously, telomerase must be replenished. Telomerase is responsible for the de novo synthesis and maintenance of telomere repeats. In general, the expression of telomerase is low or absent in most human somatic cells. Telomerase is principally located in activated lymphocytes, germ cells, and so on (Norman and Ronald, 2004).

3.3.2 Telomere and Telomerase in MSCs

Progressive telomere shortening with every cell division eventually triggers an alteration in telomere structure. When the length of telomere is reduced to a critical point, a signal is given to stop further cell division, the hallmark of cellular senescence. In contrast, cells that constitutively express telomerase can continue to divide almost indefinitely (Susan and Jhon, 2006). Counter and colleagues had reported that transfected normal human embryonic kidney cells with Simian virus 40 tumor antigen (SV40T) could express proteins of tumor virus and thus extend the lifespan of cultured cells (Dahse et al, 1997). With regard to senescence, telomere structure appears at least as important to telomere function as absolute telomere length (Norman and Ronald, 2004). From the perspective of senescence and apoptosis, the most important result of this telomere dysfunction is that the unprotected telomere end basically becomes a double-stranded break of DNA. The lifespan of cells may be regulated by multiple factors. Telomere length is a useful predictor of the residual proliferative capacity of cells (Dahse et al, 1997). Studies showed that the loss of telomere sequences because of an end replication problem might explicate a possible role in regulating cellular lifespan. Telomere shortening acts in similar fashion to a mitotic clock, counting the number of cell divisions and limiting endless proliferation. Because the lost sequences of the telomeres at each replication cycle can be resynthesized by telomerase, the enzyme has possible functions in cell immortalization.

MSCs are thought to be promising tools in cell and gene therapy. MSCs are multipotent cells with many potential clinical applications due to their capacity to be expanded *ex vivo* and to differentiate into several lineages, including osteocytes, chondrocytes, myocytes and adipocytes. However, rapid aging in MSCs *ex vivo* expansion compromise their proliferative capacity and clinical use. This limited growth potential is associated with preservation of the karyotype, telomerase activity and telomere length (Leri et al, 2005). Previous studies have demonstrated that MSCs would undergo quick telomere shortening during expansion. MSCs are capable of maintaining a normal karyotype when proliferating *ex vivo*.

Like other cell types, MSCs senescence is associated with telomere shortening during *in vitro* expansion. The range of the mean telomere length varied between 10.2 kbp to 7.8 kbp in different bone marrow samples and in different passages. Mean telomere length has an average of 9.19 kbp in the first passage, and mean telomere length 8.75 kbp by the 9th passage (Benab et al, 2006). Jesper Graakjaer and colleagues had reported the dynamic pattern of the telomere length in telomerase immortalized human MSCs (hMSCs-telo1). These cells were tested for the presence of both the endogenous and ectopic *hTERT* gene by RT-PCR. The results showed only ectopic *hTERT* gene expression was detected. TRAP assay analysis showed a high level of telomerase activity in hMSCs-telo1 (Graakjaer et al, 2007). A clear correlation between the proliferation properties of MSCs and telomere length by telomere length analysis has been suggested by Baxter and colleagues (Baxter et al, 2004). As found in other cell lines, MSCs can lose telomeres at every cell division. Once telomere length reaches a threshold of around 10 kbp in

MSCs, which is higher than those in other cell types (Roura et al, 2006), MSCs will cease cell division. Roura and colleagues assessed the senescence of human CD105 positive MSCs by telomere length assays and lipofuscin accumulation, evaluated the pluripotent differentiation by adipogenic or osteogenic inducers, and compared the myocardial phenotype in differentiated cells with cardiomyocytes. The results showed that age does not influence the adipogenic or myogenic differentiation potential of human CD105 positive MSCs (Daniel et al, 2005). MSCs and cancer stem cells share certain features such as self-renewal and differentiation potential. Actually, telomerase activity is undetectable in human MSCs both at the beginning of culture and at the passage stages during cell expansion. MSCs' telomere loss might be associated with their decreased proliferation and differentiation potentials. In general, human cells immortalize at low frequency and seem resistant to spontaneous transformation. However, Daniel Rubio had reported that MSCs in long-term culture would immortalize at high frequency and undergo spontaneous transformation (Rubio et al, 2005). He demonstrated that human adipose tissue-derived MSCs, under long-term culture conditions, once entering old age, spontaneously transform into small, clustered aggregations displaying molecular and chromosomal changes and abnormalities at a rate of about 50% (John, 1998). Other studies indicated that there was no significance in telomerase activities of MSCs at Passage 1~3 or Passage 4~7. Another study implied that embryonic stem cells could express telomerase and were functionally immortal (John, 1998). Thereby, MSCs have a different biological property of telomere compared to other adult stem cells, and have been reported to be highly resistant to transformation. The similarities between stem cell and cancer stem cell genetic programs gives rise to a proposal that some cancer stem cells could derive from human adult stem cells. Burns had reported that the long-term culture of an adult stem cell could induce a cellular autonomy capable of forming rapidly growing tumors. This concept is still controversial and requires further study.

With the development of tissue and cell engineering, scientists have paid more attention to stem cell differentiation. Studies of telomeres and telomerase are crucial to the biological characteristics of stem cell differentiation, self-renewal and proliferation, since they could affect stem cell survival.

3.4 Multilineage Transdifferentiation of MSCs

MSCs are a rare group of nonhematopoietic multipotent stem cells present in bone marrow stroma (<0.01% of the bone marrow mononuclear cell fraction). These cells are capable of differentiating into multiple mesoderm-type cells, such as osteoblasts, chondrocytes, adipocytes and fibroblasts. They contribute to the regeneration of mesenchymal tissue such as bone, cartilage, muscle, ligament, tendon and adipose. Under certain *in vitro* culture conditions, they can also differentiate into ectoderm-type cells, e.g., neuron-like cells (Dezawa et al, 2004; Black et al, 2000) and endoderm-like cells, e.g., hepatocytes (Chien et al, 2004). They have the ability to expand many times in culture while retaining their growth and multilineage potential. With their versatile growth and differentiation potential, MSCs are regarded as an ideal candidate for treating a variety of degenerative and age-related diseases for which no specific or effective treatment is currently available.

Most of our current understanding is derived from bone marrow-derived MSCs. However, MSCs similar in biological characteristics to those derived from bone marrow have been isolated from other organs, including adipose tissue (Gronthos et al, 2001; Krampera et al, 2007a; Hoogduijn et al, 2007), peripheral blood (Kuznetsov et al, 2001), umbilical cord blood (Covas et al, 2003), spleen and thymus (Krampera et al, 2003, 2007b; Hoogduijn et al, 2007), synovial membranes (De et al, 2001), lung (in't Anker et al, 2003), liver (in't Anker et al, 2003; Campagnoli et al, 2001), dental pulp (Gronthos et al, 2000; Otaki et al, 2007) and deciduous teeth (Miura et al, 2003).

MSCs were first identified for their ability to differentiate into bone and adipocytes. The classic method for MSC differentiation into osteoblasts *in vitro* is incubating MSCs with ascorbic acid, β-glycerophosphate and dexamethasone. To promote adipogenic differentiation, MSCs are incubated with dexamethasone, insulin, isobutyl methyl xanthine and indomethacin.

It has also been demonstrated that, when treated with 5-azacytidine and amphotericin B, MSCs can transdifferentiate into myoblasts that fuse into rhythmically beating myotubes (Wakitani et al, 1995). Chondrogenesis can be induced by culturing MSCs in micromass pellets in the presence of a defined medium that includes dexamethasone and transforming growth factor-beta (TGF-β) (Mackay et al, 1998).

3.4.1 MSCs and Cardiomyogenesis

A number of experimental studies have indicated that bone marrow-derived MSCs have the potential to differentiate into functional cardiomyocytes both *in vivo* and *in vitro*. There is evidence that MSCs can express cardiomyocyte markers *in vitro* when cultured in the presence of the DNA demethylating agent, 5-azacytidine.

In 1995, Wakitani (Wakitani et al, 1995) first exposed rat bone marrow-derived MSCs to 5-azacytidine for 24 hours. Long, multinucleated myotubes were observed 7∼11 days later. Cells containing Sudan black-positive droplets in their cytoplasm were also observed. Their observations provide support for the suggestion that MSCs in the bone marrow of postnatal organisms may provide a source for myoprogenitor cells, which could function in clinically relevant myogenic regeneration.

Makino (Makino et al, 1999) later isolated a cardiomyogenic (CMG) cell line from murine bone marrow stromal cells. These cells showed a fibroblast-like morphology, but the morphology changed after 5-azacytidine treatment in approximately 30% of the cells; they connected with adjoining cells after one week, formed myotube-like structures, began spontaneously beating after two weeks, and beated synchronously after three weeks. They expressed atrial natriuretic peptide and brain natriuretic peptide, and were stained with anti-myosin, anti-desmin and anti-actinin antibodies. Electron microscopy revealed a cardiomyocyte-like ultrastructure, including typical sarcomeres, a centrally positioned nucleus and atrial granules. These cells have several types of action potentials, such as sinus node-like and ventricular cell-like action potentials. All cells have a long action potential duration or plateau, a relatively shallow resting membrane potential, and a pacemaker-like late diastolic slow depolarization. Analysis of the isoform of contractile protein genes, such as myosin heavy chain, myosin light chain and alpha-actin, indicated that their muscle phenotype were similar to that of fetal ventricular cardiomyocytes. These cells express *Nkx 2.5/Csx*, *GATA4*, *TEF-1*, and *MEF-2C* mRNA before 5-azacytidine treatment and expressed *MEF-2A* and *MEF-2D* after treatment. This new cell line provides a powerful model for the study of cardiomyocyte differentiation.

Subsequent studies by Fukuda and Hakuno (Fukuda, 2001; Hakuno et al, 2002) confirmed that cardio myocytes could be differentiated from bone marrow MSCs *in vitro* by 5-azacytidine treatment. CMG cells had already expressed α_{1A}-, α_{1B}- and α_{1D}-adrenergic receptor mRNA before 5-azacytidine treatment, whereas expression of β_1-, β_2-adrenergic and M_1-, M_2-muscarinic receptors was first detected on day 1. Their findings indicate that CMG cells expressed α_{1A}-, α_{1B}- and α_{1D}-adrenergic receptor before differentiation and expressed β_1-, β_2- adrenergic and M_1-, M_2-muscarinic receptors after they obtained the cardio-myocyte phenotyps. These receptors have functional signal transduction pathways and could modulate cell function.

Bone marrow stromal cells (BMSCs) have the potential to differentiate into various cells and can transdifferentiate into myocytes if an appropriate cellular environment is provided. In Xu's study (Xu et al, 2004), they showed that BMSCs differentiation is dependent on the communication with cells in their microenvironment. BMSCs were isolated from green fluorescent protein (GFP) transgenic mice and cocultured with myocytes in a ratio of 1:40. Myocytes were obtained from ventricles of neonatal rats. Before coculturing, the BMSCs were negative for alpha-actin and exhibited a nucleus with many nuclei. After 7-day co-culture with myocytes, some BMSCs became alpha-actinin positive and formed gap junctions with native myocytes. However, BMSCs separated from myocytes by a semipermeable membrane were still negative for alpha-actinin. They concluded that BMSCs cocultured with myocytes could transdifferentiate into cells with a cardiac phenotype. The transdifferentiation processes rely on the intercellular communication of BMSCs with myocytes.

Others reported the differentiation of human adipose tissue stem cells (ATSCs) to take on cardiomyocyte properties following transient exposure to a rat cardiomyocyte extract (Gaustad et al, 2004), suggesting that cell extracts may also prove useful for investigating the molecular mechanisms of stem cell differentiation.

Animal studies *in vivo* also suggested that MSCs could differentiate into cardiomyocytes and improve cardiac function, which is attracting the attention of investigators (Tomita et al, 1999; Orlic et al, 2001a; Nagaya et al, 2005; Shake et al, 2002; Kawada et al, 2004), although most studies suggest that differentiation is extremely rare under physiological conditions.

Toma (Toma et al, 2002) investigated the potential of human MSCs from adult bone marrow to undergo myogenic differentiation once transplanted into the adult murine myocardium. A limited number of cells survived past 1 week and over time morphologically resembled the surrounding host cardiomyocytes. Immuno histochemistry revealed de novo expression of desmin, beta-myosin heavy chain, alpha-actinin, cardiac troponin T and phospholamban at levels comparable to those of the host cardiomyocytes; sarcomeric organization of the contractile proteins was observed. The purified human MSCs from adult bone marrow engrafted in the myocardium appeared to differentiate into cardiomyocytes. The persistence of the engrafted human MSCs and their *in situ* differentiation in the heart may represent the basis for using these adult stem cells for cellular cardiomyoplasty.

MSCs can differentiate into endothelial cells or smooth muscle cells in a specific microenvironment (Nagaya et al, 2005; Galmiche et al, 1993; Silva et al, 2005; Gojo et al, 2003). Angiogenesis is one of the putative mechanisms in cardiac functional recovery after myocardial infarction and stem cell transplantation, which may limit the extension of infarction and enhance repair processes. However, this also appears to be a rare event (Silva et al, 2005). The mechanisms responsible for the beneficial effects of MSCs on cardiac function are still unclear. The traditional theory holds that transplantation of MSCs into the pathological heart attenuates cardiac dysfunction by inducing cardiomyogenesis. Although a number of experimental studies reported that bone marrow-derived adult MSCs could indeed differentiate into functional cardiomyocytes both *in vivo* and *in vitro*, this concept was challenged by the finding that the differentiation of injected MSCs into cardiomyocytes is a rare event and also it has been suggested that fusion of injected MSCs with the host cardiomyocytes may occur. Murry and colleagues (Murry et al, 2004) had found that no transdifferentiation of hematopoietic stem cells into cardiomyocytes was detectable using genetic techniques to follow the cell fate, and stem-cell-engrafted hearts showed no overt increase in the numbers of cardiomyocytes compared to sham-engrafted hearts. These results indicate that hematopoietic stem cells do not readily acquire a cardiac phenotype, and raise a cautionary note for clinical studies of cellular repair in infarcted myocardium.

To test whether cellular fusion of MSCs plays a determinant role in cardiac repair, Noiseux and colleagues injected MSCs expressing Cre recombinase, with or without *Akt* (an anti-apoptotic gene), into *Cre* reporter mice (Noiseux et al, 2006). In these mice, *LacZ* is expressed only after Cre-mediated excision of a loxP-flanked stop signal and is indicative of fusion. MSCs fusion with cardiomyocytes was observed as early as 3 days at a low frequency, while a low rate of MSCs differentiated into cardiomyocytes.

3.4.2 Differentiation Fate of MSCs

Although MSCs are attractive candidate cells for therapeutic application in cardiovascular disease, some concerns have not been identified well. The most important one is that MSCs have the potential to differentiate into other mesenchymal lineages, most notably bone and fat tissue. Indeed, formation of ectopic bone/heterotopic ossification, as well as the occurrence of "fat tumors" in hematopoietic stem cell therapy, has been recognized for a long time. Yoon had found intramyocardial ossification in rats infarcted heart after injection of whole bone marrow cells, but not selected bone marrow-derived multipotent stem cells (Yoon et al, 2004). Breitbach reported recently that encapsulated structures were found in the infarcted areas of a large fraction of hearts after injected MSCs purified from bone marrow of the transgenic mice (22 of 43, 51.2%) or unfractionated bone marrow cells (6 of 46, 13.0%) (Breitbach et al, 2007). These formations contained calcifications and/or ossifications. In contrast, no pathological abnormalities were found after injection of purified hematopoietic progenitors (0 of 5, 0.0%), fibroblasts (0 of 5, 0.0%), vehicle only (0 of 30, 0.0%), or cytokine-induced mobilization of bone marrow cells (0 of 35, 0.0%). The developmental fate of bone marrow-derived cells is not restricted by the surrounding tissue after myocardial infarction and the MSC fraction underlies the extended bone formation in the infarcted myocardium. These findings seriously question the biological basis and clinical safety of using whole bone marrow and in particular MSCs, to treat non-hematopoietic disorders. At present, the importance of the transgenic nature of these cells is unclear. Taken together, these results suggest that the whole bone marrow may contain factors that stimulate bone formation in the recipient hearts.

MSCs also have the potential to differentiate into adipocytes. Although this issue has not been reported after administration into human hearts, it may have been overlooked. In a study seeking to determine whether intrarenal injection of rat MSCs could preserve the renal function in a progressive rat model of glomerulonephritis (Kunter et al, 2007), researchers found that the early beneficial effects of MSCs preserving damaged glomeruli and maintaining renal function were offset by a long-term partial mal-differentiation of intraglomerular MSCs into adipocytes accompanied by glomerular sclerosis. These data suggest that MSCs treatment can be a valuable therapeutic approach only if adipogenic mal-differentiation is prevented.

Strategies to prevent intramyocardial differentiation of injected MSCs towards unwanted cell types such as bone, cartilage or fat include *ex vivo* or *in situ* stimulation of MSCs differentiation with various factors or genes. Ideally, such stimulation of the cells simultaneously increases their therapeutic potential, while limiting their differentiation into unwanted cell types. Bartunek and colleagues reported that *ex vivo* stimulation of autologous MSCs with growth factors including bFGF, IGF-1, and bone morphogenetic protein-2 (BMP-2) prior to injection in a chronic myocardial infarction dog model caused expression of cardiomyocyte-specific genes in the MSCs, as well as a better contractile performance of treated hearts as compared to the controls treated with unstimulated MSCs (Bartunek et al, 2007). An alternative approach to drive differentiation of therapeutic cells is *ex vivo* gene therapy, as shown by van Tuyn (van Tuyn et al, 2005), who introduced the myocardiogenic transcription factor myocardin into MSCs. This led to the expression of a wide panel of cardiac genes as well as smooth muscle genes, which endowed the cells with a partial cardiomyocyte phenotype. Chemical factors, including 5-azacytidine (Wakitani et al, 1995; Makino et al, 1999; Hakuno et al, 2002) and a mixed ester of hyaluronan with butyric and retinoic acid (Ventura et al, 2007) can also enhance cardiomyogenic differentiation. Such compounds, however, act randomly on the genome, potentially resulting in variable differentiation efficiency or even deleterious effects. Engraftment of genetically modified MSCs co-overexpressing Ang-1 and Akt produced long-term histological and functional benefits in an infarcted heart (Shujia et al, 2008).

The identification of specific regulatory genes and signaling pathways that govern unique MSCs differentiation lineages remains a challenge. The domination of biological effectors to maintain a desired differentiation program or prevent disadvantageous differentiation of MSCs is necessary for effective clinical application, as in tissue engineering and regeneration.

3.5 Immunological Characteristics of MSCs

To date, MSCs are the most well characterized adult stem cells and have emerged as a promising tool in the treatment of ischemic heart diseases. Great interest has recently focused on the observation that MSCs have the ability to modulate immune responses both *in vitro* and *in vivo*. While MSCs have long been known as universal donors for transplantation, whether allogeneic or xenogeneic, recent studies have shown that MSCs may have immunogenicity properties and elicit immune rejection. Therefore, MSCs may constitute a previously unrecognized part of the immune system and may play a dual functional role. The immunological characteristics and immuno-modulatory functions of MSCs and their possible mechanisms of action will be discussed in this section.

3.5.1 Immunological Characteristics of MSCs

Recent data from *in vitro* studies has demonstrated that MSCs can evade immune surveillance and modulate immune responses. This may be due to the cell surface molecules of MSCs. MSCs express intermediate levels of human leukocyte antigen (HLA) major histocompatibility (MHC) Class I molecules and almost no MHC Class II molecule expression is detected on the cell surface (Tse et al, 2003; Di et al, 2002). Le Blanc and colleague found that MHC II molecules were present intracellularly by western-blot analysis and over 90% of MSCs expressed MHC Class II on the cell surface after induction by interferon-γ (Le et al, 2003). However, even following the upregulation of MHC molecules on the cell surface, MSCs still failed to elicit proliferation of allogeneic lymphocytes in a co-culture system (Tse et al, 2003; Di et al, 2002; Le et al, 2003; Krampera et al, 2003). MSCs also do not express Fas ligand or costimulatory molecules, such as B7-1, B7-2, CD40, and $CD40_L$, all of which play a role in immune evasion and immune modulation (Majumdar et al, 2003). A large number of studies have shown that MSCs can modulate T cell, B cell proliferation and activation, dendritic cell maturation and function, and can result in immune suppression *in vitro* and *in vivo*. These pave the way for clinical application of MSCs transplantation between allogeneic individuals.

However, recent studies have demonstrated that allogeneic MSCs infused into MHC-mismatched mice were sometimes rejected. A challenge to the concept of MSCs immunoprivilege exists, which suggests that MSCs are not intrinsically immunoprivileged and cannot serve as a "universal donor" in immunocompetent MHC-mismatched recipients (Eliopoulos et al, 2005; Nauta et al, 2006). Additionally, IL-2-activated natural killer (NK) cells are able to efficiently kill allogeneic and autologous MSCs due to surface ligands that were recognized by NK receptors and the low levels of MHC I expression (Spaggiari et al, 2006). Furthermore, MSCs were shown to perhaps function as antigen-presenting cells (APCs) (Chan et al, 2006).

3.5.1.1 MSCs and T Lymphocytes

T lymphocytes, also known as T cells, play an important role in human immunity. A variety of studies have focused on this issue to investigate the immunomodulatory effects of MSCs.

3.5.1.1.1 MSCs Suppress T Cell Proliferation

As early as 1998, Klyushnenkova reported that human MSCs suppressed allogeneic T cell responses *in vitro* (Klyushnenkova et al, 2005). Since then, an increasing amount of data has been generated regarding the immunomodulatory characteristics of MSCs. Many groups have demonstrated *in vitro* that cultured MSCs have the ability to suppress T cell proliferation induced by allogeneic peripheral blood mononuclear cells (PBMCs), allogeneic splenocytes, mitogens (phyto-hemagglutinin, concanavalin A) and anti-CD3/anti-CD28 antibodies (Tse et al, 2003; Di et al, 2002; Le et al, 2003; Krampera et al, 2003; Djouad et al, 2003; Aggarwal and Pittenger, 2005; Maccario et al, 2005). Additionally, MSCs from placenta (Li et al, 2007), adipose (Keyser et al, 2007), and even spleen and thymus (Krampera et al, 2007b) have demonstrated a suppressive effect on T lymphocytes. Interestingly, even after osteogenic induction *in vitro*, bone marrow and adipose-derived MSCs still retain their inhibitory effect on T cells (Niemeyer et al, 2007). However, the mechanisms underlying this effect are largely unknown.

3.5.1.1.2 Probable Mechanisms

- Induction of T cell anergy
  T cell anergy is a hyporesponsive state in which the lymphocyte is intrinsically functionally inactivated in the presence of an antigen. Anergic T cells lose the ability of proliferation and cytokine production is reduced in response to antigenic stimulation as a result of insufficient costimulation (Schwartz, 2003). MSCs that lack expression of costimulatory molecules induce T lymphocyte anergy (Zappia et al, 2005). Generally, an anergic state can be overcome by the addition of exogenous IL-2 (Schwartz, 2003). However, Glennie and collaborators demonstrated that allogeneic MSCs rendered T cells anergic and removal of MSCs restored IFN-γ production, but not T cell proliferation, in mixed lymphocyte cultures, despite the exogenous addition of IL-2. MSC-mediated T cell arrest in G_0/G_1 phase of the cell cycle occurred by irreversible inhibition of the cyclin D_2 expression and upregulation of $p27^{Kip1}$ expression (Glennie et al, 2005). G_0/G_1 cell-cycle arrest was confirmed and the $p16^{INK4A}$-cyclin D_1/ cdk4 and $p21^{waf1}$, $p27^{kip1}$-cyclin E/cdk2 complex pathway were all implicated in the mechanism (Kim et al, 2007).
- Induction of regulatory T cells
  The regulatory T cells play a pivotal role in suppression of immune responses, especially in autoimmune pathologies. Several studies indicated that the interaction of MSCs and lymphocytes increased the number of $CD4^+$ and $CD25^+$ regulatory T cells, favored Foxp3 and CTLA4 expression, and displayed a suppressive function on other T lymphocyte subpopulations (Maccario et al, 2005; Li et al, 2007; Meisel et al, 2004). Another study showed that depletion of $CD25^+$ cells from the purified $CD4^+$ T cells did not prevent MSC-mediated inhibition (Beyth et al, 2005). Further insight into the function of regulatory T cells indicated that $CD4^+$ and $CD8^+$ regulatory T cells generated in co-cultures of PBMCs and MSCs may amplify the reported immunosuppressive effect that is mediated by MSCs (Prevosto et al, 2007).
- Soluble factors
  Many studies have shown that the immunomodulatory effect of MSCs is

mediated by soluble factors. Both transforming growth factor-β (TGF-β) and hepatocyte growth factor (HGF) have been investigated. Di Nicola and coworkers showed that neutralization of TGF-β_1 or HGF increased a minimal BMSC-suppressed T lymphocyte proliferation, while simultaneous inhibition of the two cytokines restored the proliferation of T cells (Di et al, 2002). Other studies confirmed the result of exclusion as a single role for TGF-β in MSCs-induced immunosuppression (Tse et al, 2003; Krampera et al, 2003; Beyth et al, 2005).

Indoleamine 2,3-dioxygenase (IDO) catalyzes the conversion of tryptophan to kynurenine and active IDO results in reduced lymphocyte proliferation (Nasef et al, 2007). Meisel and collaborators reported that MSCs expressed IDO protein and exhibited functional IDO activity after stimulation by IFN-γ. Their results indicated that IDO-mediated tryptophan depletion can act as a T cell inhibitory effector mechanism in human MSCs (Meisel et al, 2004). In contrast, a different study showed that suppression was not substantially reversed by addition of either extra tryptophan or IDO inhibitor (Tse et al, 2003). Therefore, a partial and probable role of IDO in the immunomodulatory effect of MSCs is agreed upon by a majority of researchers (Krampera et al, 2006).

Prostaglandin E_2 (PGE_2) production has been found to be increased in the co-culture of MSCs and PBMCs (Aggarwal and Pittenger, 2005), yet the effect of PGE_2 on MSC-induced immune suppression is contradictory. In the system of co-culture of MSCs and PBMCs stimulated with anti-CD3/CD28 antibodies, inhibition of PGE_2 production resulted in no restored proliferation (Tse et al, 2003). However, mitogen-activated PBMCs co-cultured with MSCs could restore the proliferation through inhibition of PGE_2 synthesis (Glennie et al, 2005).

Other factors, such as IL-10 (Beyth et al, 2005), nitric oxide (NO) (Sato et al, 2007), HLA-G (Nasef et al, 2007), and stromal cell-derived factor 1 (SDF-1) (Le et al, 2004b), have shown some effects on MSCs induced suppression. However, controversy still remains. One explanation is that the effect of different soluble factors on MSCs induced immune suppression is dependent on the type of stimuli received by MSCs (e.g., allogeneic determinants, membrane-bound proteins, mitogens, cytokines, etc.).

- Cell contact-dependent mechanism

  A few studies have demonstrated that contact-dependent mechanisms are implicated in MSCs immunogenicity. Krampera showed that the MSCs inhibitory effect required cell contact and the inhibitory activity was abrogated when MSCs were added to the T cell cultures in a Transwell system or when MSCs were replaced by MSCs culture supernatant (Krampera et al, 2003). The Augello group confirmed this data and showed that the B7-H1/PD-1 pathway was involved in the mechanism (Augello et al, 2005).

3.5.1.2 MSCs and B Cells

MSCs also exhibit an inhibitory effect on B lymphocytes. The proliferation of splenic B cells stimulated with anti-CD40 monoclonal antibody was greatly inhibited by MSCs to the same degree as the inhibition observed in T cells (Glennie et al, 2005). Other groups have also obtained similar results. After coronary artery ligation at different timepoints, Weimin and colleagues demonstrated that MSCs could effectively suppress the proliferation of B cells in a concentration of 1:5 (MSCs/B cells) and 1:10, whereas a stimulating effect was observed at 1:100 (which could be due to their own hyperreactivity); the inhibitory effect was dose-dependent (Deng et al, 2005). Furthermore, maximum suppression was observed in the ratio of 1:1 and disappeared in the ratios of 5:1 and 10:1 in another study (Corcione et al, 2006). This result differs greatly from that of T cells that have been shown to be dose-dependent (Djouad et al, 2003). This may indicate that the concentration of 1:1 is a critical point; a lower concentration is dose-dependent, and a higher dose may not be. MSCs also have the ability to decrease B cell activation and immunoglobin secretion (Deng et al, 2005; Corcione et al, 2006). Similar to T cells, Corcione and colleagues demonstrated that B cell proliferation was inhibited by MSCs through an arrest in the G_0/G_1 phase of the cell cycle, while independent of apoptosis. As indicated by transwell experiments, soluble factors produced by MSCs were found to be a major mechanism of B cell suppression. They also found the CXCR4, CXCR5, and CCR7 chemokine receptors of B cells were significantly down regulated by MSCs. This suggested a significant inhibition after coronary artery ligation on migration in response to the given chemokines, which finally affected the function (Corcione et al, 2006).

3.5.1.3 MSCs and APCs

Dendritic cells (DCs) are the most potent antigen-presenting cells that are specialized in antigen uptake, transportation and presentation. They play a role in initiating cell-mediated immunity (Banchereau et al, 2000). Many studies have shown that MSCs have the ability to modulate differentiation, maturation and the function of DCs.

Differentiation of DCs is inhibited by MSCs. In 2004 Zhang and collaborators showed that MSCs inhibited monocyte-derived DC differentiation, while MSC supernatant did not (Zhang et al, 2004). Later, Jiang and coinvestigators confirmed the suppressive mechanism of direct cell contact. They further found that suppression of DCs differentiation can also be in a contact-independent manner at a higher MSC/monocyte ratio in a transwell system (Jiang et al, 2005). Differentiation of $CD34^+$ and bone marrow derived DCs was also inhibited in recent studies (Chen, 2006; Jung et al, 2007).

Maturation of DCs is suppressed by MSCs. MSCs have been found to suppress upregulation of APC related molecules, including HLA-DR, CD40, CD80, CD86, as well as the maturation marker CD83, during the process of

DC maturation (Maccario et al, 2005; Beyth et al, 2005; Sotiropoulou et al, 2006). Intriguingly, the co-culture of mature DCs with MSCs resulted in a significant decrease in HLA-DR, CD1a, and co-stimulatory molecules CD80 and CD86, which indicated MSCs could reverse the mature DCs into an immature phenotype (Jiang et al, 2005).

MSCs affect the function of DCs. Zhang and colleagues showed that endocytosis of monocyte-derived DCs was inhibited by MSCs and MSCs supernatant, and the ability to stimulate T lymphocyte proliferation was also restricted (Zhang et al, 2004). With a newly developed time-lapse video microscopic technique, Jung and coworkers demonstrated that matured DCs actively migrated directionally in response to a powerful DCs-attracting chemokine, CCL21, whereas the MSCs co-cultured DCs did not (Jung et al, 2007). More recently, English and colleagues showed MSCs interfere in antigen presentation by DCs and prevent dendritic cell migration ability to CCL19 (English et al, 2008).

The mechanisms involved in the inhibitory effect may include cell contact and soluble factors. Many groups have implicated IFN-γ, TNF-α, PGE_2, IL-6, IL-10 and IL-12 in playing roles in the MSC-induced DC suppression (Aggarwal and Pittenger, 2005; Beyth et al, 2005; Jiang et al, 2005; Chen et al, 2007). However, the specific mechanisms are not clearly defined.

3.5.1.4 MSCs and NK Cells

NK cells play a crucial role in innate immunity and are known to display strong cytolytic activity against tumor or virus-infected cells. NK cells express activating and inhibitory receptors and the balance between them determines the function by which NK cells kill targets. Protection from NK cell-mediated cytotoxicity occurs when MHC Class I molecules bind to NK cell inhibitory receptors. NK cells are the major source of IFN-γ in the process of immune response (Biron, 1997; Yoon et al, 2007).

Spaggiari reported that MSCs prevented the proliferation of resting NK cells in response to IL-2 or IL-15 at all NK/MSC ratios ranging from 1:1 to 8:1 (Spaggiari et al, 2006). On the other hand, only partial inhibition of proliferation of pre-activated NK cells by IL-2 could be detected. Intriguingly, they showed at the same time that MSCs express a broad range of surface ligands recognized by activating NK receptors, which resulted in the cells being highly susceptible to NK cell-mediated lysis. The study demonstrated that autologous and allogeneic MSCs could be efficiently lysed by IL-2-activated NK cells that produced IFN-γ, whereas freshly isolated NK cells could not, even at high NK/MSCs ratios. Furthermore, they studied the effect of NK cells on MSCs after upregulated expression of MHC Class I by IFN-γ treatment. Surprisingly, MSCs were less susceptible to NK cell-mediated lysis and failed to induce IFN-γ production by NK cells. Taken together, these data indicate IFN-γ is a potent modulator of MSC/NK cell crosstalk (Spaggiari et al, 2006). Similar results were obtained by Sotiropoulou and co-investigators (Sotiropoulou et al, 2006).

3.5.2 *In vivo* Studies

Although MSCs look prominsing in the modulation of immune responses *in vitro*, controversy still remains in *in vivo* studies. In 2002 Bartholomew and coinvestigators showed for the first time that intravenous injection of bone marrow-derived MSCs could prolong the survival of allogeneic skin graft in baboons (Bartholomew et al, 2002). Later on, Djouad confirmed the similar beneficial effect of MSCs without rejection in immunocompetent mice (Djouad et al, 2003). They also demonstrated that although allogeneic MSCs could engraft and bone formation was observed in immunocompetent mice, lymphocytic infiltration was seen at the periphery of the newly formed bone and inside the cartilaginous matrix. The study concluded that allogeneic MSCs elicited an immune response, yet the allogeneic bone was not rejected.

In addition, MSCs have also been proposed as a treatment for autoimmune diseases (van Laar and Tyndall, 2006). In the model of multiple sclerosis (MS), it was shown that intravenous administration of MSCs can ameliorate encephalomyelitis (EAE). Administration the onset of the disease and at the peak of the disease, but not after the disease, resulted in stabilization and decreased inflammatory infiltration and demyelination (Zappia et al, 2005). Similar results were recently obtained which confirm the enhancing effect (Gerdoni et al, 2007). Augello reported that a single injection of allogeneic MSCs prevented the occurrence of severe, irreversible damage to bone and cartilage in collagen-induced arthritis, a mouse model for human rheumatoid arthritis (Augello et al, 2007). However, MSCs did not confer any benefit in the same model for another group (Djouad et al, 2005). Combination of allogeneic MSCs and sex-mismatched bone marrow cells (BMCs) helped to normalize blood glucose and serum insulin concentrations in a type 1 diabetes model, while both BMCs and MSCs alone were ineffective. B cell-specific T lymphocytes from a diabetic pancreas disappeared after MSC injection, indicating that MSCs inhibit T cell-mediated immune responses which, in turn, are able to survive in this altered immunological milieu (Urban et al, 2008).

In addition, MSC infusion was found to promote the success of the clinical outcome following hematopoietic stem cell transplantation (HSCT) (Koc et al, 2000). MSCs may become a useful approach in HSCT since results from Phase I clinical trials support the feasibility and safety (Lazarus et al, 1995). Most intriguingly, Le Blanc and coworkers demonstrated that injection of haplo-identical MSCs associated with an immunosuppressive treatment improved the clinical outcome in a patient with severe treatment-resistant grade IV acute graft-versus-host disease (GVHD) of the gut and liver (Le et al, 2004a). Many studies involving a substantial number of patients have supported the idea that MSCs represent a valuable option for allogeneic HSCT recipients suffering from acute GVHD (Lazarus et al, 2005; Maitra et al, 2004).

However, Nauta reported that the addition of recipient-derived MSCs to the MHC-mismatched BMCs promoted the engraftment, whereas hampered engraftment was observed by the addition of allogeneic donor derived MSCs. They also found a memory T cell response triggered by the infusion of allogeneic MSCs (Nauta et al, 2006). Allogeneic treatment of MSCs elicited an increased proportion of host-derived lymphoid $CD8^+$, natural killer T (NKT) and NK infiltrating cells compared with syngeneic controls in mice (Eliopoulos et al, 2005). This data suggests that MSCs are not intrinsically immunoprivileged.

3.5.3 Immune-related Properties of MSCs in Cardiology

Similar to the aforementioned *in vivo* studies, the results of MSCs allogeneic or xenogeneic transplantation in cardiology are conflicting. Saito and coworkers showed that xenogeneic marrow stromal cells from C57BL/6 mice survived in the recipient rats for at least 13 weeks after transplantation without any immunosuppression. Numerous mouse cells were found in the infarcted myocardium after coronary artery ligation at different timepoints, suggesting migration. Subsequently, MSCs survival and differentiation were detected in the peri-infarct site (Saito et al, 2002). Our own data demonstrated that allogeneic MSCs transplantation to the infarcted myocardium could improve the heart function and with no obvious immune rejection observed (Wang et al, 2004).

However, Grinnemo and colleagues used human MSCs for transplantation into rat infarcted myocardium and found that MSCs could only be identified in the myocardium of immunodeficient rats. They also detected significant myocardial infiltration of round cells, mostly macrophages, in the area of injection, while this reaction was less intense in immunodeficient rats (Grinnemo et al, 2004). More recently, allogeneic MSCs transplanted into the ischemic heart were unfortunately found to elicit immune responses *in vivo* (Poncelet et al, 2007).

Much has been accomplished in the investigation of MSCs in recent years. MSCs have been shown to play an important role in immune modulation both *in vitro* and *in vivo*. There are some important issues that should receive particular attention and warrant further investigation. First, the safety of MSC application in immune diseases should be taken into account. Given that MSCs are immunosuppressive, the stimulation of tumor growth by MSCs, rather than inhibition, might be the result of direct effects on malignant cells or suppression of anti-tumor immune responses (Djouad et al, 2003). Secondly, contradictory results still exist, especially in *in vivo* studies; the immune modulation effect and definite mechanisms of MSCs are still unknown. In-depth studies of MSCs in immune regulation are necessary and urgent in the future to ensure the successful and safe use of MSCs in clinical therapies.

3.6 Conclusion

In summary, MSCs, as stem cells, prossess a property of indefinite proliferation, which is associated with unique structures of telomeres and telomerase. MSCs express a multitude of surface receptors and produce a variety of cardioprotective signalling molecules, and have the ability to differentiate into both myoccyte and vascular lineages. Various ion channels exist on MSCs, contributing to their electrophysiological functions, including the electrometrical coupling with host cardiomyocytes. The multi-lineage potential of MSCs, in combination with their immunoprivileged status, make MSCs a promising source for cell therapy in cardiac diseases.

References

Aggarwal S, Pittenger MF (2005) Human mesenchymal stem cells modulate allogeneic immune cell responses. Blood, 105(4):1815-1822

Augello A, Tasso R, Negrini SM, Amateis A, Indiveri F, Cancedda R, Pennesi G (2005) Bone marrow mesenchymal progenitor cells inhibit lymphocyte proliferation by activation of the programmed death 1 pathway. Eur J Immunol, 35(5):1482-1490

Augello A, Tasso R, Negrini SM, Cancedda R, Pennesi G (2007) Cell therapy using allogeneic bone marrow mesenchymal stem cells prevents tissue damage in collagen-induced arthritis. Arthritis Rheum, 56(4):1175-1186

Aussmus B, Schächinger V, Teupe C, Britten M, Lehmann R, Dóbert N, Grunwald F, Aicher A, Urbich C, Martin H, Hoelzer D, Dimmeler S, Zeiher AM (2002) Transplantation of progenitor cells and regeneration enhancement in acute myocardial infarction (TOPCARE-AMI). Circulation, 106(24):3009-3017

Ball SG, Shuttleworth CA, Kielty CM (2007) Mesenchymal stem cells and neovascularization: role of platelet-derived growth factor receptors. J Cell Mol Med, 11(5):1012-1030

Banchereau J, Briere F, Caux C, Davoust J, Lebecque S, Liu YJ, Pulendran B, Palucka K (2000) Immunobiology of dendritic cells. Annu Rev Immunol, 18:767-811

Barry FP, Boynton RE, Haynesworth S, Murphy JM, Zaia J (1999) The monoclonal antibody SH-2, raised against human mesenchymal stem cells, recognizes an epitope on endoglin (CD105). Biochem Biophys Res Commun, 265(1):134-139

Bartholomew A, Sturgeon C, Siatskas M, Ferrer K, McIntosh K, Patil S, Hardy W, Devine S, Ucker D, Deans R, Moseley A, Hoffman R (2002) Mesenchymal stem cells suppress lymphocyte proliferation *in vitro* and prolong skin graft survival *in vivo*. Exp Hematol, 30(1):42-48

Bartunek J, Croissant JD, Wijns W, Gofflot S, de Lavareille A, Vanderheyden M, Kaluzhny Y, Mazouz N, Willemsen P, Penicka M, Mathieu M, Homsy C,

De Bruyne B, McEntee K, Lee IW, Heyndrickx GR (2007) Pretreatment of adult bone marrow mesenchymal stem cells with cardiomyogenic growth factors and repair of the chronically infarcted myocardium. Am J Physiol Heart Circ Physiol, 292(2):H 1095-1104

Baxter MA, Wynn RF, Jowitt SN, Wraith JE, Fairbairn LJ, Bellantuono I(2004) Study of telomere length reveals rapid aging of human marrow stromal cells following *in vitro* expansion. Stem Cells, 22(5):675-682

Beyth S, Borovsky Z, Mevorach D, Liebergall M, Gazit Z, Aslan H, Galun E, Rachmilewitz J (2005) Human mesenchymal stem cells alter antigen-presenting cell maturation and induce T-cell unresponsiveness. Blood, 105(5):2214-2219

Biron CA (1997) Activation and function of natural killer cell responses during viral infections. Curr Opin Immunol, 9(1):24-34

Black IB, Woodbury D (2000) Adult rat and human bone marrow stromal cells differentiate into neurons. J Neurosci Res, 61(4):364-370

Bonab MM, Alimoghaddam K, Talebian F, Ghaffari SH, Ghavamzadeh A, Nikbin B (2006) Aging of mesenchymal stem cell *in vitro*. BMC Cell Biol, 7:14

Breitbach M, Bostani T, Roell W, Xia Y, Dewald O, Nygren JM, Fries JW, Tiemann K, Bohlen H, Hescheler J, Welz A, Bloch W, Jacobsen SE, Fleischmann BK (2007) Potential risks of bone marrow cell transplantation into infarcted hearts. Blood, 110 (4):1362-1369

Caddick J, Kingham PJ, Gardiner NJ, Wiberg M, Terenghi G (2006) Phenotypic and functional characteristics of mesenchymal stem cells differentiated along a Schwann cell lineage. Glia, 54(8):840-849

Campagnoli C, Roberts IA, Kumar S, Bennett PR, Bellantuono I, Fisk NM (2001) Identification of mesenchymal stem/progenitor cells in human first-trimester fetal blood, liver and bone marrow. Blood, 98(8):2396-2402

Chan JL, Tang KC, Patel AP, Bonilla LM, Pierobon N, Ponzio NM, Rameshwar P (2006) Antigen-presenting property of mesenchymal stem cells occurs during a narrow window at low levels of interferon-gamma. Blood, 107(12):4817-4824

Chang MG, Tung L, Sekar RB, Chang CY, Cysyk J, Dong PH, Marban E, Abraham MR (2006) Proarrhythmic potential of mesenchymal stem cell transplantation revealed in an *in vitro* coculture model. Circulation, 113(15):1832-1841

Chen M, Fan ZC, Liu XQ, Zhang L, Rao L, Yang Q, Huang DJ (2005) Changes of myocardial electrophysiology after stem cell transplantation. Chin J Cardiac Pacing Electrophysiol, 19(2):124-127

Chen L, Zhang W, Yue H, Han Q, Chen B, Shi M, Li J, Li B, You S, Shi Y, Zhao RC (2007) Effects of human mesenchymal stem cells on the differentiation of dendritic cells from $CD34^+$ cells. Stem Cells Dev, 16(5):719-732

Chien CC, Yen BL, Lee FK, Lai TH, Chen YC, Chan SH, Huang HI (2004) *In vitro* hepatic differentiation of human mesenchymal stem cells. Hepatology, 40(6):1275-1284

Chiou MY, Xu, Longaker MT (2006) Mitogenic and chondrogenic effects of fibroblast growth factor-2 in adipose-derived mesenchymal cells. Biochem Biophys Res Commun, 343(2):644-652

Cohen IS, Rosen AB, Gaudette GR (2007) A Caveat Emptor for myocardial regeneration: mechanical without electrical recovery will not suffice. J Mol Cell Cardiol, 42(2):285-288

Cong YS, Wright WE, Shay JW (2002) Human telomerase and its regulation. Microbiol Mol Biol Rev, 66(3):407-425

Corcione A, Benvenuto F, Ferretti E, Giunti D, Cappiello V, Cazzanti F, Risso M, Gualandi F, Mancardi GL, Pistoia V, Uccelli A (2006) Human mesenchymal stem cells modulate B-cell functions. Blood, 107(1):367-372

Covas DT, Siufi JL, Silva AR, Orellana MD (2003) Isolation and culture of umbilical vein mesenchymal stem cells. Braz J Med Biol Res, 36(9):1179-1183

Dahse R, Fiedler W, Ernst G (1997) Telomeres and telomerase: biological and clinical importance. Clinical Chemistry, 43(5):708-714

De Bari C, Dell'Accio F, Tylzanowski P, Luyten FP (2001) Multipotent mesenchymal stem cells from adult human synovial membrane. Arthritis Rheum, 44(8):1928-1942

Deng W, Han Q, Liao L, You S, Deng H, Zhao RC (2005) Effects of allogeneic bone marrow-derived mesenchymal stem cells on T and B lymphocytes from BXSB mice. DNA Cell Biol, 24(7):458-463

Dezawa M, Kanno H, Hoshino M, Cho H, Matsumoto N, Itokazu Y, Tajima N, Yamada H, Sawada H, Ishikawa H (2004) Specific induction of neuronal cells from bone marrow stromal cells and application for autologous transplantation. J Clin Invest,113 (12):1701-1710

Di Nicola M, Carlo-Stella C, Magni M, Milanesi M, Longoni PD, Matteucci P, Grisanti S, Gianni AM (2002) Human bone marrow stromal cells suppress T-lymphocyte proliferation induced by cellular or nonspecific mitogenic stimuli. Blood, 99(10):3838-3843

Djouad F, Plence P, Bony C, Tropel P, Apparailly F, Sany J, Noel D, Jorgensen C (2003) Immunosuppressive effect of mesenchymal stem cells favors tumor growth in allogeneic animals. Blood, 102(10):3837-3844

Djouad F, Fritz V, Apparailly F, Louis-Plence P, Bony C, Sany J, Jorgensen C, Noel D (2005) Reversal of the immunosuppressive properties of mesenchymal stem cells by tumor necrosis factor alpha in collagen-induced arthritis. Arthritis Rheum, 52(5):1595-1603

Djouad F, Delorme B, Maurice M, Bony C, Apparailly F, Louis-Plence P, Canovas F, Charbord P, Noel D, Jorgensen C (2007) Microenvironmental changes during differentiation of mesenchymal stem cells towards chondrocytes. Arthritis Res Ther, 9(2):R33

Dominici M, Le Blanc K, Mueller I, Slaper-Cortenbach I, Marini F, Krause D, Deans R, Keating A, Prockop Dj, Horwitz E (2006) Minimal criteria for defining multipotent mesenchymal stromal cells. The International Society for Cellular Therapy position statement. Cytotherapy, 8(4):315-317

Eliopoulos N, Stagg J, Lejeune L, Pommey S, Galipeau J (2005) Allogeneic marrow stromal cells are immune rejected by MHC Class I- and Class II-mismatched recipient mice. Blood,106(13):4057-4065

English K, Barry FP, Mahon BP (2008) Murine mesenchymal stem cells suppress dendritic cell migration, maturation and antigen presentation. Immunol Lett, 115(1):50-58

Erices A, Conget P, Rojas C, Minguell JJ (2002) Gp130 activation by soluble interleukin-6 receptor/interleukin-6 enhances osteoblastic differentiation of human bone marrow-derived mesenchymal stem cells. Exp Cell Res, 280(1):24-32

Falconi D, Oizumi K, Aubin JE (2007) Leukemia inhibitory factor influences the fate choice of mesenchymal progenitor cells. Stem Cells, 25(2):305-312

Fukuda K (2001) Development of regenerative cardiomyocytes from mesenchymal stem cells for cardiovascular tissue engineering. Artif Organs, 5(3):187-193

Gagari E, Rand MK, Tayari L, Vastardis H, Sharma P, Hauschka PV, Damoulis PD (2006) Expression of stem cell factor and its receptor, c-kit, in human oral mesenchymal cells. Eur J Oral Sci, 114(5):409-415

Galmiche MC, Koteliansky VE, Brière J, Hervé P, Charbord P (1993) Stromal cells from human long-term marrow cultures are mesenchymal cells that differentiate following a vascular smooth muscle differentiation pathway. Blood, 82(1):66-76

Gang EJ, Jeong JA, Han S, Yan Q, Jeon CJ, Kim H (2006) *In vitro* endothelial potential of human UC blood-derived mesenchymal stem cells. Cytotherapy, 8(3):215-227

Gaustad KG, Boquest AC, Anderson BE, Gerdes AM, Collas P (2004) Differentiation of human adipose tissue stem cells using extracts of rat cardiomyocytes. Biochem Biophys Res Commun, 314(2):420-427

Gerdoni E, Gallo B, Casazza S, Musio S, Bonanni I, Pedemonte E, Mantegazza R, Frassoni F, Mancardi G, Pedotti R, Uccelli A (2007) Mesenchymal stem cells effectively modulate pathogenic immune response in experimental autoimmune encephalomyelitis. Ann Neurol, 61(3):219-227

Glennie S, Soeiro I, Dyson PJ, Lam EW, Dazzi F (2005) Bone marrow mesenchymal stem cells induce division arrest anergy of activated T cells. Blood,105(7): 2821-2827

Gnecchi M, He H, Noiseux N, Liang OD, Zhang L, Morello F, Mu H, Melo LG, Pratt RE, Ingwall JS, Dzau VJ (2006) Evidence supporting paracrine hypothesis for Akt-modified mesenchymal stem cell-mediated cardiac protection and functional improvement. Faseb J, 20(6):661-669

Gojo S, Gojo N, Takeda Y, Mori T, Abe H, Kyo S, Hata J, Umezawa A (2003) *In vivo* cardiovasculogenesis by direct injection of isolated adult mesenchymal stem cells. Exp Cell Res, 288(1):51-59

Graakjaer J, Christensen R, Kolvraa S, Serakinci N (2007) Mesenchymal stem cells with high telomerase expression do not actively restore their chromosome arm specific telomere length pattern after exposure to ionizing radiation. BMC Mol Biol, 13(8): 49

Grinnemo KH, Mansson A, Dellgren G, Klingberg D, Wardell E, Drvota V, Tammik C, Holgersson J, Ringden O, Sylven C, Le Blanc K (2004) Xenoreactivity and engraftment of human mesenchymal stem cells transplanted into infarcted rat myocardium. J Thorac Cardiovasc Surg, 127(5):1293-1300

Gronthos S, Mankani M, Brahim J, Robey PG, Shi S (2000) Postnatal human dental pulp stem cells (DPSCs) *in vitro* and *in vivo.* Proc Natl Acad Sci USA, 97 (25):13625-13630

Gronthos S, Franklin DM, Leddy HA, Robey PG, Storms RW, Gimble JM (2001) Surface protein characterization of human adipose tissue-derived stromal cells. J Cell Physiol, 189(1):54-63

Hakuno D, Fukuda K, Makino S, Konishi F, Tomita Y, Manabe T, Suzuki Y, Umezawa A, Ogawa S (2002) Bone marrow-derived regenerated cardiomyocytes

(CMG Cells) express functional adrenergic and muscarinic receptors. Circulation, 105(3):380-386

Heubach JF, Graf EM, Leutheuser J, Bock M, Balana B, Zahanich I, Christ T, Boxberger S, Wettwer E, Ravens U (2003) Electrophysiological properties of human mesenchymal stem cells. J Physiol, 554(3):659-672

Honczarenko M, Le Y, Swierkowski M, Ghiran I, Glodek AM, Silberstein LE (2006) Human bone marrow stromal cells express a distinct set of biologically functional chemokine receptors. Stem Cells, 24(4):1030-1041

Hoogduijn MJ, Crop MJ, Peeters AM, Van Osch GJ, Balk AH, Ijzermans JN, Weimar W, Baan CC (2007) Human heart, spleen, and perirenal fat-derived mesenchymal stem cells have immunomodulatory capacities. Stem Cells Dev, 16(4):597-604

in't Anker PS, Noort WA, Scherjon SA, Kleijburg-van der Kear C, Kruisselbrink AB, van Bezooijen RL, Beekhuizen W, Willemze R, Kanhai HH, Fibbe WE (2003) Mesenchymal stem cells in human second-trimester bone marrow, liver, lung and spleen exhibit a similar immunophenotype but a heterogeneous multilineage differentiation potential. Haematologica, 88(8): 845-852

Ip JE, Wu Y, Huang J, Zhang L, Pratt RE, Dzau VJ (2007) Mesenchymal stem cells use integrin beta1 not CXC chemokine receptor 4 for myocardial migration and engraftment. Mol Biol Cell, 18(8):2873-2882

Jiang XX, Zhang Y, Liu B, Zhang SX, Wu Y, Yu XD, Mao N (2005) Human mesenchymal stem cells inhibit differentiation and function of monocyte-derived dendritic cells. Blood, 105(10):4120-4126

John MS (1998) Can ends justify the means? Telomeres and the mechanisms of replicative senescence and immortalization in mammalian cells. Proc Natl Acad Sci USA, 95(16):9078-9081

Jones EA, English A, Henshaw K, Kinsey SE, Markham AF, Emery P, McGonagle D (2004) Enumeration and phenotypic characterization of synovial fluid multipotential mesenchymal progenitor cells in inflammatory and degenerative arthritis. Arthritis Rheum, 50(3):817-827

Jootar S, Pornprasertsud N, Petvises S, Rerkamnuaychoke B, Disthabanchong S, Pakakasama S, Ungkanont A, Hongeng S (2006) Bone marrow derived mesenchymal stem cells from chronic myeloid leukemia t(9;22) patients are devoid of Philadelphia chromosome and support cord blood stem cell expansion. Leuk Res, 30(12): 1493-1498

Jung YJ, Ju SY, Yoo ES, Cho SJ, Cho KA, Woo SY, Seoh JY, Park JW, Han HS, Ryu KH (2007) MSC-DC interactions: MSC inhibit maturation and migration of BM-derived DC. Cytotherapy, 9(5):451-458

Kawada H, Fujita J, Kinjo K, Matsuzaki Y, Tsuma M, Miyatake H, Muguruma Y, Tsuboi K, Itabashi Y, Ikeda Y, Ogawa S, Okano H, Hotta T, Ando K, Fukuda K (2004) Nonhematopoietic mesenchymal stem cells can be mobilized and differentiate into cardiomyocytes after myocardial infarction. Blood, 104(12):3581-3587

Kawano S, Shoji S, Ichinose S, Yamagata K, Tagami M, Hiraoka M (2002) Characterization of Ca^{2+} signaling pathways in human mesenchymal stem cells. Cell Calcium, 32(4):165-174

Keyser KA, Beagles KE, Kiem HP (2007) Comparison of mesenchymal stem cells from different tissues to suppress T-cell activation. Cell Transplant, 16(5):555-562

Kim JA, Hong S, Lee B, Hong JW, Kwak JY, Cho S, Kim CC (2007) The inhibition of T-cells proliferation by mouse mesenchymal stem cells through the induction of p16INK4A-cyclin D1/cdk4 and p21waf1, p27kip1-cyclin E/cdk2 pathways. Cell Immunol, 245(1):16-23

Klyushnenkova E, Mosca JD, Zernetkina V, Majumdar MK, Beggs KJ, Simonetti DW, Deans RJ, McIntosh KR (2005) T cell responses to allogeneic human mesenchymal stem cells: immunogenicity, tolerance, and suppression. J Biomed Sci, 12(1):47-57

Koc ON, Gerson SL, Cooper BW, Dyhouse SM, Haynesworth SE, Caplan AI, Lazarus HM (2000) Rapid hematopoietic recovery after coinfusion of autologous-blood stem cells and culture-expanded marrow mesenchymal stem cells in advanced breast cancer patients receiving high-dose chemotherapy. J Clin Oncol, 18(2):307-316

Krampera M, Glennie S, Dyson J, Scott D, Laylor R, Simpson E, Dazzi F (2003) Bone marrow mesenchymal stem cells inhibit the response of naive and memory antigen-specific T cells to their cognate peptide. Blood, 101(9):3722-3729

Krampera M, Pasini A, Rigo A, Scupoli MT, Tecchio C, Malpeli G, Scarpa A, Dazzi F, Pizzolo G, Vinante F (2005) HB-EGF/HER-1 signaling in bone marrow mesenchymal stem cells: inducing cell expansion and reversibly preventing multilineage differentiation. Blood, 106(1):59-66

Krampera M, Cosmi L, Angeli R, Pasini A, Liotta F, Andreini A, Santarlasci V, Mazzinghi B, Pizzolo G, Vinante F, Romagnani P, Maggi E, Romagnani S, Annunziato F (2006) Role for interferon-gamma in the immunomodulatory activity of human bone marrow mesenchymal stem cells. Stem Cells, 24(2):386-398

Krampera M, Marconi S, Pasini A, Gali M, Rigotti G, Mosna F, Tinelli M, Lovato L, Anghileri E, Andreini A, Pizzolo G, Sbarbati A, Bonetti B (2007a) Induction of neural-like differentiation in human mesenchymal stem cells derived from bone marrow, fat, spleen and thymus. Bone, 40(2): 382 -390

Krampera M, Sartoris S, Liotta F, Pasini A, Angeli R, Cosmi L, Andreini A, Mosna F, Bonetti B, Rebellato E, Testi MG, Frosali F, Pizzolo G, Tridente G, Maggi E, Romagnani S, Annunziato F (2007b) Immune regulation by mesenchymal stem cells derived from adult spleen and thymus. Stem Cells Dev, 16(5):797-810

Kunter U, Rong S, Boor P, Eitner F, Müller-Newen G, Djuric Z, van Roeyen CR, Konieczny A, Ostendorf T, Villa L, Milovanceva-Popovska M, Kerjaschki D, Floege J (2007b) Mesenchymal stem cells prevent progressive experimental renal failure but maldifferentiate into glomerular adipocytes. J Am Soc Nephrol, 18(6):1754-1764

Kuznetsov SA, Mankani MH, Gronthos S, Satomura K, Bianco P, Robey PG (2001) Circulating skeletal stem cells. J Cell Biol, 153(5):1133-1140

Lazarus HM, Haynesworth SE, Gerson SL, Rosenthal NS, Caplan AI (1995) *Ex vivo* expansion and subsequent infusion of human bone marrow-derived stromal progenitor cells (mesenchymal progenitor cells): implications for therapeutic use. Bone Marrow Transplant, 16(4):557-564

Lazarus HM, Koc ON, Devine SM, Curtin P, Maziarz RT, Holland HK, Shpall EJ, McCarthy P, Atkinson K, Cooper BW, Gerson SL, Laughlin MJ, Loberiza FR, Jr, Moseley AB, Bacigalupo A (2005) Cotransplantation of HLA-identical sibling culture-expanded mesenchymal stem cells and hematopoietic stem cells in hematologic malignancy patients. Biol Blood Marrow Transplant, 11(5):389-398

Le Blanc K, Tammik C, Rosendahl K, Zetterberg E, Ringden O (2003) HLA expression and immunologic properties of differentiated and undifferentiated mesenchymal stem cells. Exp Hematol, 31(10):890-896

Le Blanc K, Rasmusson I, Sundberg B, Gotherstrom C, Hassan M, Uzunel M, Ringden O (2004a) Treatment of severe acute graft-versus-host disease with third party haploidentical mesenchymal stem cells. Lancet, 363(9419):1439-1441

Le Blanc K, Rasmusson I, Gotherstrom C, Seidel C, Sundberg B, Sundin M, Rosendahl K, Tammik C, Ringden O (2004b) Mesenchymal stem cells inhibit the expression of CD25 (interleukin-2 receptor) and CD38 on phytohaemagglutinin-activated lymphocytes. Scand J Immunol, 60(3):307-315

Leri A, Kajstura J, Anversa P (2005) Cardiac stem cells and mechanisms of myocardial regeneration. Physiol Rev., 85(4):1373-1416

Li C, Zhang W, Jiang X, Mao N (2007) Human-placenta-derived mesenchymal stem cells inhibit proliferation and function of allogeneic immune cells. Cell Tissue Res, 330(3):437-446

Li GR, Sun HY, Deng XL, Lau CP (2005) Characterization of ionic currents in human mesenchymal stem cells from bone marrow. Stem Cells, 23(3):371-382

Li TS, Hamano K, Suzuki K, Ito H, Zempo N, Matsuzaki M (2002) Improved angiogenic potency by implantation of *ex vivo* hypoxia prestimulated bone marrow cells in rats. Am J Physiol Heart Circ Physiol, 283(2):H468-473

Lisignoli G, Cristino S, Piacentini A, Cavallo C, Caplan AI, Facchini A (2006) Hyaluronan-based polymer scaffold modulates the expression of inflammatory and degradative factors in mesenchymal stem cells: Involvement of Cd44 and Cd54. J Cell Physiol, 207(2):364-373

Maccario R, Podesta M, Moretta A, Cometa A, Comoli P, Montagna D, Daudt L, Ibatici A, Piaggio G, Pozzi S, Frassoni F, Locatelli F (2005) Interaction of human mesenchymal stem cells with cells involved in alloantigen-specific immune response favors the differentiation of $CD4^+$ T-cell subsets expressing a regulatory/suppressive phenotype. Haematologica, 90(4):516-525

Mackay AM, Beck SC, Murphy JM, Barry FP, Chichester CO, Pittenger MF (1998) Chondrogenic differentiation of cultured human mesenchymal stem cells from marrow. Tissue Eng, 4(4):415-428

Maitra B, Szekely E, Gjini K, Laughlin MJ, Dennis J, Haynesworth SE, Koc ON (2004) Human mesenchymal stem cells support unrelated donor hematopoietic stem cells and suppress T-cell activation. Bone Marrow Transplant, 33(6):597-604

Majumdar MK, Keane-Moore M, Buyaner D, Hardy WB, Moorman MA, McIntosh KR, Mosca JD (2003) Characterization and functionality of cell surface molecules on human mesenchymal stem cells. J Biomed Sci, 10(2):228-241

Makino S, Fukuda K, Miyoshi S, Konishi F, Kodama H, Pan J, Sano M, Takahashi T, Hori S, Abe H, Hata J, Umezawa A, Ogawa S (1999) Cardiomyocytes can be generated from marrow stromal cells *in vitro*. J Clin Invest, 103(5):697-705

Mareschi K, Novara M, Rustichelli D, Ferrero I, Guido D, Carbone E, Medico E, Madon E, Vercelli A, Fagioli F (2006) Neural differentiation of human mesenchymal stem cells: Evidence for expression of neural markers and eag K^+ channel types. Exp Hematol, 34(11):1563-1572

Meeker AK, Hicks JL, Iacobuzio-Donahue CA, Montgomery EA, Westra WH, Chan TY, Ronnett BM, De Marzo AM (2004) Telomere length abnormalities occur early in the initiation of epithelial carcinogenesis. Clinical Cancer Research, 10(10): 3317-3326

Meisel R, Zibert A, Laryea M, Gobel U, Daubener W, Dilloo D (2004) Human bone marrow stromal cells inhibit allogeneic T-cell responses by indoleamine 2,3-dioxygenase -mediated tryptophan degradation. Blood, 103(12):4619-4621

Mills WR, Mal N, Kiedrowski MJ, Unger R, Forudi F, Popovic ZB, Penn MS, Laurita KR (2007) Stem cell therapy enhances electrical viability in myocardial infarction. J Mol Cell Cardiol, 42(2):304-314

Miura M, Gronthos S, Zhao M, Lu B, Fisher LW, Robey PG, Shi S (2003) stem cells from human exfoliated deciduous teeth. Proc Natl Acad Sci USA, 100(10): 5807-5812

Moon HJ, Jeon ES, Kim YM, Lee MJ, Oh CK, Kim JH (2007) Sphingosylphosphorylcholine stimulates expression of fibronectin through TGF-beta1-Smad-dependent mechanism in human mesenchymal stem cells. Int J Biochem Cell Biol, 39(6):1224-1234

Murry CE, Soonpaa MH, Reinecke H, Nakajima H, Nakajima HO, Rubart M, Pasumarthi KB, Virag JI, Bartelmez SH, Poppa V, Bradford G, Dowell JD, Williams DA, Field LJ (2004) Haematopoietic stem cells do not transdifferentiate into cardiac myocytes in myocardial infarcts. Nature, 428(6983):664-668

Nagaya N, Kangawa K, Itoh T, Iwase T, Murakami S, Miyahara Y, Fujii T, Uematsu M, Ohgushi H, Yamagishi M, Tokudome T, Mori H, Miyatake K, Kitamura S (2005) Transplantation of mesenchymal stem cells improves cardiac function in a rat model of dilated cardiomyopathy. Circulation, 112(8):1128-1135

Nasef A, Mathieu N, Chapel A, Frick J, Francois S, Mazurier C, Boutarfa A, Bouchet S, Gorin NC, Thierry D, Fouillard L (2007) Immunosuppressive effects of mesenchymal stem cells: involvement of HLA-G. Transplantation, 84(2): 231-237

Nauta AJ, Westerhuis G, Kruisselbrink AB, Lurvink EG, Willemze R, Fibbe WE (2006) Donor-derived mesenchymal stem cells are immunogenic in an allogeneic host and stimulate donor graft rejection in a nonmyeloablative setting. Blood,108(6): 2114-2120

Niemeyer P, Kornacker M, Mehlhorn A, Seckinger A, Vohrer J, Schmal H, Kasten P, Eckstein V, Sudkamp NP, Krause U (2007) Comparison of immunological properties of bone marrow stromal cells and adipose tissue-derived stem cells before and after osteogenic differentiation *in vitro*. Tissue Eng, 13(1):111-121

Noiseux N, Gnecchi M, Lopez-Ilasaca M, Zhang L, Solomon SD, Deb A, Dzau VJ, Pratt RE (2006) Mesenchymal stem cells overexpressing Akt dramatically repair infarcted myocardium and improve cardiac function despite infrequent cellular fusion or differentiation. Mol Ther, 14(6): 840-850

Norman ES, Ronald AD (2004) Telomeres, stem cells, senescence, and cancer. J Clin Invest, 113(2):160-168

Orlic D, Kajstura J, Chimenti S, Bodine DM, Leri A, Anversa P (2001a) Bone marrow cells regenerate infarcted myocardium. Nature, 410(6829):701-705

Orlic D, Kajstura J, Chimenti S, Limana F, Jakoniuk I, Quaini F, Nadal-Ginard B, Bodine DM, Leri A, Anversa P (2001b) Mobilized bone marrow cells repair the infarcted heart improving function and survival. Proc Natl Acad Sci USA, 98: 10344-10349

Ortiz LA, Dutreil M, Fattman C, Pandey AC, Torres G, Go K, Phinney DG (2007) Interleukin 1 receptor antagonist mediates the antiinflammatory and antifibrotic effect of mesenchymal stem cells during lung injury. Proc Natl Acad Sci USA, 104(26): 11002-11007

Otaki S, Ueshima S, Shiraishi K, Sugiyama K, Hamada S, Yorimoto M, Matsuo O (2007) Mesenchymal progenitor cells in adult human dental pulp and their ability to form bone when transplanted into immunocompromised mice. Cell Biol Int, 31(10):1191-1197

Peiffer I, Eid P, Barbet R, Li ML, Oostendorp RA, Haydont V, Monier MN, Milon L, Fortunel N, Charbord P, Tovey M, Hatzfeld J, Hatzfeld A (2007) A sub-population of high proliferative potential-quiescent human mesenchymal stem cells is under the reversible control of interferon alpha/beta. Leukemia, 21(4):714-724

Pijnappels DA, Schalij MJ, van Tuyn JV, Ypey DL, de Vries AA, van der Wall EE, van der Laarse A, Atsma DE (2006) Progressive increase in conduction velocity across human mesenchymal stem cells is mediated by enhanced electrical coupling. Cardiovas Res, 72(2): 282-291

Poncelet AJ, Vercruysse J, Saliez A, Gianello P (2007) Although pig allogeneic mesenchymal stem cells are not immunogenic *in vitro*, intracardiac injection elicits an immune response *in vivo*. Transplantation, 83(6):783-790

Potapova I, Plotnikov A, Lu ZJ, Danilo P, Valiunas V, Qu JH, Doronin S, Zuckerman J, Shlapakova IN, Gao JY, Pan ZM. Herron AJ, Rovinson RB, Brink PR, Rosen MR, Cohen IS (2004) Human mesenchymal stem cells as gene delivery system to create cardiac pacemakers. Cir Res, 94(7):952-959

Prevosto C, Zancolli M, Canevali P, Zocchi MR, Poggi A (2007) Generation of $CD4^+$ or $CD8^+$ regulatory T cells upon mesenchymal stem cell-lymphocyte interaction. Haematologica, 92(7):881-888

Ren XQ, Pu JL, Zhang S, Jiang YH, Wu GZ, Meng L, Wang FZ (2005) Cardiac atrioventricular conduct function improved by autologous transplantation of mesenchymal stem cells in canine atrioventricular conduct block model. Chin J Cardiac Pacing Electrophysiol, 19(1):48-52

Risbud MV, Albert TJ, Guttapalli A, Vresilovic EJ, Hillibrand AS, Vaccaro AR, Shapiro IM (2004) Differentiation of mesenchymal stem cells towards a nucleus pulposus-like phenotype *in vitro*: implications for cell-based transplantation therapy. Spine, 29(23):2627-2632

Roura S, Farré J, Soler-Botija C, Llach A, Hove-Madsen L, Cairó J, Gòdia F, Cinca J, Bayes-Genis A (2006) Effect of aging on the pluripotential capacity of human $CD105^+$ mesenchymal stem cells. Eur J Heart Fail, 8(6):555-563

Rubio D, Garcia-Castro J, Martín MC, de la Fuente R, Cigudosa JC, Lloyd A, Bernad A (2005) Spontaneous Human Adult Stem Cell Transformation. Cancer Research, 65(11): 3035-3039

Saito T, Kuang JQ, Bittira B, Al-Khaldi A, Chiu RC (2002) Xenotransplant cardiac chimera: immune tolerance of adult stem cells. Ann Thorac Surg, 74(1):19-24

Sato K, Ozaki K, Oh I, Meguro A, Hatanaka K, Nagai T, Muroi K, Ozawa K (2007) Nitric oxide plays a critical role in suppression of T-cell proliferation by mesenchymal stem cells. Blood, 109(1):228-234

Schächinger V, Erbs S, Elsasser A, Haberbosch W, Hambrecht R, Holschermann H, Yu J, Corti R, Mathey DG, Hamm CW, Suselbeck T, Assmus B, Tonn T, Dimmeler S, Zeiher AM (2006) Improved clinical outcome after intracoromary administration of bone marrow derived progenitor cells in acute myocardial infarction: final 1-year results of the REPAIR-AMI trial. Eur Heart J, 27(23):2775-2783

Schwartz RH (2003) T cell anergy. Ann Rev Immunol, 21:305-334

Shake JG, Gruber PJ, Baumgartner WA, Senechal G, Meyers J, Redmond JM, Pittenger MF, Martin BJ (2002) Mesenchymal stem cell implantation in a swine myocardial infarct model: engraftment and functional effects. Ann Thorac Surg, 73(6): 1919-1925

Shay JW, Wright WE (2005) Senescence and immortalization: role of telomeres and telomerase. Carcinogenesis, 26(5):867-874

Shujia J, Haider HK, Idris NM, Lu G, Ashraf M (2008) Stable therapeutic effects of mesenchymal stem cell-based multiple gene delivery for cardiac repair. Cardiovasc Res, 77(3):525-533

Silva WA Jr, Covas DT, Panepucci RA, Proto-Siqueira R, Siufi JL, Zanette DL, Santos AR, Zago MA (2003) The profile of gene expression of human marrow mesenchymal stem cells. Stem Cells, 21(6):661-669

Silva GV, Litovsky S, Assad JA, Sousa AL, Martin BJ, Vela D, Coulter SC, Lin J, Ober J, Vaughn WK, Branco RV, Oliveira EM, He R, Geng YJ, Willerson JT, Perin EC (2005) Mesenchymal stem cells differentiate into an endothelial phenotype, enhance vascular density, and improve heart function in a canine chronic ischemia model. Circulation, 111(2):150-156

Sotiropoulou PA, Perez SA, Gritzapis AD, Baxevanis CN, Papamichail M (2006) Interactions between human mesenchymal stem cells and natural killer cells. Stem Cells, 24(1):74-85

Spaggiari GM, Capobianco A, Becchetti S, Mingari MC, Moretta L (2006) Mesenchymal stem cell-natural killer cell interactions, evidence that activated NK cells are capable of killing MSCs, whereas MSCs can inhibit IL-2-induced NK-cell proliferation. Blood, 107(4):1484-1490

Susan MB, John PM (2006) Telomeres, chromosome instability and cancer. Nucleic Acids Research, 34(8):2408-2417

Toma C, Pittenger MF, Cahill KS, Byrne BJ, Kessler PD (2002) Human mesenchymal stem cells differentiate to a cardiomyocyte phenotype in the adult murine heart. Circulation, 105(1):93-98

Tomita S, Li RK, Weisel RD, Mickle DA, Kim EJ, Sakai T, Jia ZQ (1999) Autologous transplantation of bone marrow cells improves damaged heart function. Circulation, 100(19 Suppl):II247-256

Tse HF, Xue T, Lau CP, Siu CW, Wang K, Zhang QY, Tomaselli GF, Akar FG, Li RA (2006) Bioartificial sinus node constructed via *in vivo* gene transfer of an engineered pacemaker HCN Channel reduces the dependence on electronic pacemaker in a sick-sinus syndrome model. Circulation, 114(10):1000-1011

Tse WT, Pendleton JD, Beyer WM, Egalka MC, Guinan EC (2003) Suppression of allogeneic T-cell proliferation by human marrow stromal cells: implications in transplantation. Transplantation, 75(3):389-397

Uemura R, Xu M, Ahmad N, Ashraf M (2006) Bone marrow stem cells prevent left ventricular remodeling of ischemic heart through paracrine signaling. Circ Res, 98(11):1414-1421

Urbán VS, Kiss J, Kovács J, Gócza E, Vas V, Monostori E, Uher F (2008) Mesenchymal stem cells cooperate with bone marrow cells in therapy of diabetes. Stem Cells, 26(1):244-253

Ventura C, Cantoni S, Bianchi F, Lionetti V, Cavallini C, Scarlata I, Foroni L, Maioli M, Bonsi L, Alviano F, Fossati V, Bagnara GP, Pasquinelli G, Recchia FA, Perbellini A (2007) Hyaluronan mixed esters of butyric and retinoic Acid drive cardiac and endothelial fate in term placenta human mesenchymal stem cells and enhance cardiac repair in infarcted rat hearts. J Biol Chem, 282(19):14243-14252

van Laar JM, Tyndall A (2006) Adult stem cells in the treatment of autoimmune diseases. Rheumatology (Oxford), 45(10):1187-1193

van Tuyn J, Knaän-Shanzer S, van de Watering MJ, de Graaf M, van der Laarse A, Schalij MJ, van der Wall EE, de Vries AA, Atsma DE (2005) Activation of cardiac and smooth muscle-specific genes in primary human cells after forced expression of human myocardin. Cardiovasc Res, 67(2): 245-255

Wakitani S, Saito T, Caplan AI (1995) Myogenic cells derived from rat bone marrow mesenchymal stem cells exposed to 5-azacytidine. Muscle Nerve, 18(12): 1417-1426

Wang JA, Li CL, Fan YQ, He H, Sun Y (2004) Allograftic bone marrow-derived mesenchymal stem cells transplanted into heart infarcted model of rabbit to renovate infarcted heart. J Zhejiang Univ Sci, 5(10):1279-1285

Wang JA, Xie XJ, Sun Y, He H, Jiang CY, Zhou BQ, Luo RH, Dong L (2005) Autologous mesenchynml stem cells transplantation in patients with post-myocardial infarction and cardiac dysfunction. Chin J Emerg Med, 14(12):996-999

Wang JA, Luo RH, Zhang X, Xie XJ, Hu XY, He AN, Chen J, Li JH (2006a) Bone marrow mesenchymal stem cell transplantation combined with perindopril treatment attenuates infarction remodelling in a rat model of acute myocardial infarction. J Zhejiang Univ Sci B, 7(8): 641-647

Wang JA, Xie XJ, He H, Sun Y, Jiang J, Luo RH, Fan YQ, Dong L (2006b) A prospective, randomized, controlled trial of autologous mesenchymal stem cells transplantation for dilated cardiomyopathy. Zhonghua Xin Xue Guan Bing Za Zhi, 34(2):107-110

Wang PP, Wang JH, Yan ZP, Hu MY, Lau GK, Fan ST, Luk JM (2004) Expression of hepatocyte-like phenotypes in bone marrow stromal cells after HGF induction. Biochem Biophys Res Commun, 320(3):712-716

Wang S, Wang JA, Li J, Zhou J, Wang H (2008) Voltage-dependent potassium channels are involved in staurosporine-induced apoptosis of rat mesenchymal stem cells. Cell Biol Int, 32(2):312-319

Wang SP, Wang JA, Luo RH, Cui WY, Wang H (2008) Potassium channel currents in rat mesenchymal stem cells and their possible roles in cell proliferation. Clin Exp Pharmacol Physiol, 35(9):1077-1084

Xie XJ, Wang JA, Cao J, Zhang X (2006) Differentiation of bone marrow mesenchymal stem cells induced by myocardial medium under hypoxic conditions. Acta Pharmacol Sin, 27(9):1153-1158

Xu M, Wani M, Dai YS, Wang J, Yan M, Ayub A, Ashraf M (2004) Differentiation of bone marrow stromal cells into the cardiac phenotype requires intercellular communication with myocytes. Circulation, 110(17):2658-2665

Yoon YS, Park JS, Tkebuchava T, Luedeman C, Losordo DW (2004) Unexpected severe calcification after transplantation of bone marrow cells in acute myocardial infarction. Circulation, 109(25):3154-3157

Yoon SR, Chung JW, Choi I (2007) Development of natural killer cells from hematopoietic stem cells. Mol Cells, 24(1):1-8

Zappia E, Casazza S, Pedemonte E, Benvenuto F, Bonanni I, Gerdoni E, Giunti D, Ceravolo A, Cazzanti F, Frassoni F, Mancardi G, Uccelli A (2005) Mesenchymal stem cells ameliorate experimental autoimmune encephalomyelitis inducing T-cell anergy. Blood, 106(5):1755-1761

Zhang N, Li J, Wang J, Luo R, Jiang J (2008) Bone marrow mesenchymal stem cells induces angiogenesis and attenuates the remodeling of diabetic cardiomyopathy. Exp Clin Endocrinol, 116(2):104-111

Zhang W, Ge W, Li C, You S, Liao L, Han Q, Deng W, Zhao RC (2004) Effects of mesenchymal stem cells on differentiation, maturation, and function of human monocyte-derived dendritic cells. Stem Cells Dev, 13(3):263-271

Zhu H, Mitsuhashi N, Klein A, Barsky LW, Weinberg K, Barr ML, Demetriou A, Wu GD (2006) The role of the hyaluronan receptor CD44 in mesenchymal stem cell migration in the extracellular matrix. Stem Cells, 24(4):928-935

4

Utilization of MSCs for Repairing Cardiomyocytes

Xiaojie Xie[1], **Qiyuan Xu**[2]

[1,2]Second Affiliated Hospital, Zhejiang University College of Medicine, Hangzhou, China
E-mail: [1]xiaojiexie@hotmail.com
[2]aceline_qiy@hotmail.com

Abstract: Heart disease including myocardial infarction and ischemia is associated with the irreversible loss of cardiomyocytes and vasculature, both via apoptosis or necrosis. However, the native capacity for the renewal and repair of myocardial tissue is inadequate as have been current therapeutic measures to prevent left ventricular remodeling and heart failure. Cell transplantation has emerged as a potentially viable therapeutic approach to directly repopulate and repair the damaged myocardium. A detailed analysis and a vision for future progress in MSCs applications, both in myocardial infarction and cardiomyopathy are presented in this review, highlighting research cardiology.

Cardiomyocytes come from the splanchnic mesoderms mesenchymal cells. In the embryonic development period, the mesenchymal cells differentiate to myoblast cells, and on to the mature myocytes. It has not yet been clarified whether cardiac stem cells (CSCs) exist in the adult heart. Investigators in several laboratories concur with the notion that the heart contains a compartment of undifferentiated cells with the characteristics of stem cells (Hierlihy et al, 2002; Urbanek, 2003, 2005). However, the actual number of CSCs remains controversial. Reports in mice (Matsuura et al, 2004), rats (Beltrami et al, 2003), dogs (Linke et al, 2005), and humans (Hierlihy et al, 2002) indicate that there is 1 stem cell per 8,000 to 20,000 myocytes, or 32,000 to 80,000 cardiac cells.

A new conceptual framework of the heart has emerged and it is now viewed as a self-renewing organ in which myocyte regeneration occurs throughout the organism's lifespan (Goldman and Wurzel, 2001). The adult heart has a sub-population of myocytes that are not terminally differentiated; these myocytes evidently can reenter the cell cycle and undergo nuclear mitotic division soon after infarction. Although CSCs are efficient in preserving organ homeostasis and cell turnover, the decompensated heart is characterized by a loss of myocytes and vascular structures. These factors cannot be counteracted by the activation and differentiation of CSCs, which undergo progressive replicative senescence, leading to a dramatic reduction of the stem cell compartment. Cardiac aging and chronic heart failure can occur, resulting in myocardial apoptosis and necrosis. This limited proliferation and self-renewal cannot compensate for heart injury, leading to replacement of cardiomyocytes by fibroblasts and consequent formation of fibrosis. Due to scar- and ischemia-related post-infarction events, clinical manifestations are enormous and heterogeneous. The damaged left ventricle undergoes progressive "remodeling" and chamber dilation. These events reflect an apparent lack of effective intrinsic mechanisms for myocardial repair and regeneration. Unless deep (and still unknown) modifications are introduced in the area proximate to the damage to force the proliferation of resident cardiac progenitor cells, all restorative therapies must consider the use of exogenous multipotent stem cells capable to differentiate, at least, into cardiomyocytes. From this point of view, bone marrow-located stem cells have been considered to display the required biologic properties for a cell therapy approach to treat patients with myocardial infarction.

In addition to the use of bone marrow-derived hematopoietic precursor cells, cellular, molecular and preclinical data have shown that bone marrow-derived MSCs represent a suitable cell archetype for regenerative purposes after myocardial infarction. Under proper stimulation, MSCs can be induced to differentiate into myocytes, endothelium and smooth muscle cells in the infarcted heart (Kajstura et al, 2005), revealing a high degree of plasticity. MSCs isolated from several human sources, including bone marrow and peripheral and umbilical cord blood, exhibit a high *ex vivo* expansion capacity. This property has been used to assess the biologic properties of MSCs to perform transfection with viral vectors (Conget and Minguell, 2000; Partridge, 2002) and initiate studies toward the use of MSCs in clinical strategies (Horwitz et al, 1999; Barry and Murphy, 2004). The promising therapeutic effect of MSCs relies on their capacity to engraft and survive long term in distinctive target tissue.

In this review we will analyze the experimental evidence that warrants the utilization of MSCs in the treatment of myocardial infarction and chronic heat failure.

4.1 Application of MSCs on Myocardial Infarction

Myocardial Infarction (MI), over 95% of which is caused by atherosclerosis of the coronary artery, is one of the cardiovascular emergencies with high disability and mortality. Atherosclerotic plaques lead to intraluminal sclerosis and a slowing down of blood flow, contributing to cardiac ischemia and necrosis over time. This is a serious and persistent process. The complications that can occur in patients with extensive MI, such as malignant arrhythmia, heart failure, formation of ventricular aneurysm, and sudden cardiac death, are life-threatening, but can also disrupt the quality of life. Medications, percutaneous coronary intervention (PCI) and coronary artery bypass grafting (CABG) are involved in treating patients with MI, failing to induce functional cardiomyogensis, but scar formation.

Evidences concerning bone marrow stem cells repairing the infarcted myocardium has accumulated based on a multitude of animal studies. The first reports from Makino and colleagues (Makino et al, 1999) in 1999 had demonstrated that bone marrow stem cells could *in vitro* differentiate into cardiomyocytes induced by 5-azacytidine. *In vivo* evidence of transdifferentiation from Orlic studies in 2001 (Orlic et al, 2001) showed that bone marrow stem cells transplanted into the infarcted myocardium can differentiate into cardiomyocates and consequently improve cardiac function (Fig. 4.1). MSCs have also been shown as suitable candidates for MI repair. One of the famous studies in China is from Ge JB (Ma et al, 2004; Zhang et al, 2005), who established MI models in swine and Sprague-Dawley (SD) rats and injected MSCs transcoronarily or intravenously. As a result, MSC transplantation could improve the cardiac function, mediated by promoting cardiomyogenesis and neoangiogeneis in the ischemic borderline of infarcted myocardium. The increases in the ejection fraction (EF) by echocardiogram were correlated with the baseline. The worse the baseline of the ejection fraction in MI models, the better the therapeutic effect of MSCs transplantation.

We have been focusing on the therapeutic effects and safety of MSC transplantation in animal models as well as patients suffering from MI or chronic heat failure. We have established MI models in New Zealand rabbits (Wang et al, 2004, 2005), SD rats (Chen et al, 2006; Wang, 2006) and mice (Hu et al, 2007, 2008) by ligation of the left anterior descending artery respectively. Allogenic bone marrow-derived MSCs were isolated, expanded *in vitro* and analyzed by flow cytometry before transplantation. MSCs at Passage 3 to 10 were ready for transplantation and trypsinized from the plates, washed twice with sterile phosphate buffer solution (PBS), centrifuged and suspended in PBS or saline. MSCs suspension was injected intramyocardially into the

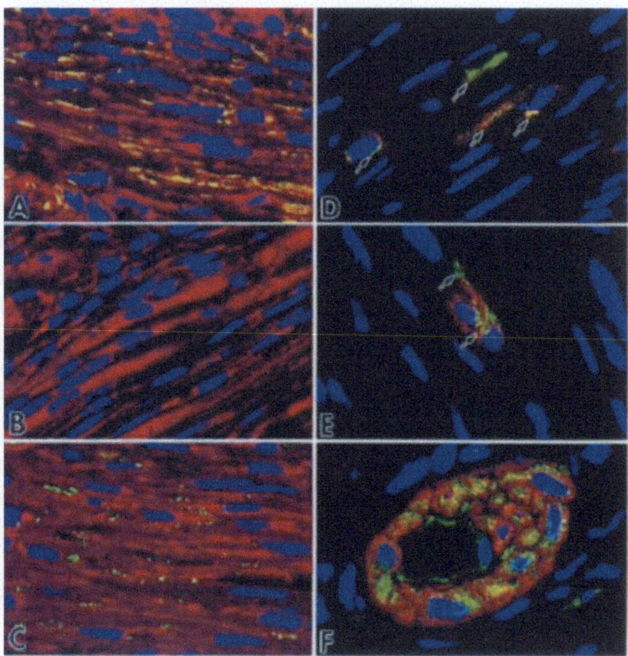

Fig. 4.1. Markers of differentiating cardiac cells. (A-F) Labeling of CM by nestin (A, yellow), desmin (B, red), and connexin 43 (C, green); red fluorescence = cardiac myosin (A and C). (D and E) Yellow-green fluorescence reflects labeling of EC by flk-1 (arrows, D) and VE-cadherin (arrows, E); red fluorescence = factor VIII in EC (D and E). (F) Green fluorescence labeling of SMC cytoplasms by flk-1; endothelial lining is also labeled by flk-1; red fluorescence = α-smooth muscle actin; blue fluorescence = propidium iodide (PI) labeling of nuclei. (A and E, ×1,200; B and F ×800; C, ×1,400; D, ×1,800.)

infarcted region and the ischemic borderline respectively. Morphological and pathophysiological parameters, including cardiac function, ventricular remodeling and the possible mechanisms, were evaluated in the engrafted heart and the controls. Consequently, compared with those in the controls, MSCs transplantation could significantly increase ejection fraction (EF) and fractional shortening (FS), decrease left ventricular internal diameter at end-diastole (LVIDd) and relieve ventricular remodeling. The therapeutic effects could also be achieved by autologous and heterogenous MSCs transplantation. Further pathological examinations showed that injected MSCs were localized in the injection sites and transdifferentiated into cardiomyocyte-like cells, endothelial cells and smooth muscle cells, thus reducing the infarcted extension and improving cardiac contractility by the survived myocytes (Wang et al, 2004, 2005, 2006; Chen et al, 2006). Our *in vitro* studies indicated that MSCs under hypoxic conditions could not only significantly synthesize and up-regulate a multitude of growth factors, including hypoxia induced factors-1 alpha (HIF-1α), vascular endothelial growth factors (VEGF), erythropoietin (EPO) and its receptor, angiotensin I, Flk-1, etc, but promote anti-apoptotic gene expression, such as Bcl-xl, Bcl-2, caspase 3. Hypoxia conditioned MSCs could enhance neoangiogenesis, alleviate apoptosis and attenuate ventricular remodeling in MI animals (Hu et al, 2008; Wang et al, 2008). The anti-apoptosis by MSCs therapy was associated with inactivation of voltage-dependent potassium channels in MSCs (Wang S et al, 2008). Post-infarcted ventricular remodeling attenuated by MSCs transplantation might be mediated by down-regulating the expressions of matrix metalloproteinases (MMP-2, MMP-9) and reducing fibrosis (Wang et al, 2006).

Endothelial progenitor cells (EPCs) are also ideal candidates for cardiac celloplasty. Human EPCs isolated from adult periperal blood were labelled and injected intravenously into athymic rats 3-hour post-MI (Kawamoto et al, 2001). EPCs immigrated into the infarcted myocardium and participated in neoangiogenesis. EPCs transplantation contributed to the improvement of cardiac function, a significant increase of capillary density in the ischemic region, and diminution of the scar area in the infarcted myocardium. Specific human endothelial markers could also be detected in these engrafted cells. In clinical trials, EPC therapy could increase left ventricular ejection fraction (LVEF) and improve the survival of infarcted cardiomyocytes in patients with MI compared with those in the control groups. The therapeutic effects of MSCs transplantation may be achieved by reconstitution of the blood supply in the infarcted myocardium (Assmus et al, 2002; Liu et al, 2005).

In summary, bone marrow cell transplantation to treat patients with MI or ischemic cardiomyopathy is safe, feasible and effective, especially with MSCs. The mechanisms of the therapeutic effects using cell transplantation might include not only stem cell transdifferentiation, but neoangiogenesis, anti-apoptosis, paracrine and so forth.

- It has been demonstrated that transplanted bone marrow-derived MSCs could transdifferentiate into cardiomyocytes-like cells, endothelium and smooth muscle cells in the infarcted myocardium (Makino et al, 1999; Orlic et al, 2001; Wang, 2004, 2005; Kajstura et al, 2005). However, there are inconsistent reports that some investigators regard the transplanted cells as cell fusion with the host cardiomyocytes rather than transdifferentiation (Alvarez-Dolado et al, 2003; Terada et al, 2002).
- Evidence showed that bone marrow-derived MSCs can secrete a plethora of growth factors, including basic fibroblast growth factor (bFGF), vascular endothelial growth factor (VEGF), interleukin-1 beta (IL-1β), and tumor necrosis factor-2 alpha (TNF-2α), etc. The paracrine effects of MSCs might contribute to neoangiogenesis and anti-apoptosis in the ischemic myocardium, improve myocardial perfusion, especially for the hibernating and stunned cardiomyocytes, which may limit the extension of the infarcted

area and protect it from ischemic injury (Hu et al, 2008; Kamihata et al, 2001).

- Another possible mechanism is that bone marrow-derived MSCs therapy could attenuate the compensatory activation of sympathetic nerves after MI, activate cardiac vagus nerve system and keep the balance of cardiac autonomic nerve regulation. MSCs transplantation might relieve the remodeling of cardiac nerves in the non-infarcted region as well (Ding et al, 2006), promoting the sprouting of cardiac nerve terminals, and thus improve the neurotrophy and neuroregulation in the infarcted myocardium (Pak et al, 2003).
- In addition, bone marrow-derived MSCs could express the proteins involved in the intercellular gap junction, including connexin 40, connexin 43 and connexin 45 in the infarcted region. The transplanted cells could establish the intercellular electric-mechanic coupling with the host cardiomyocytes, contributing to host heart contraction and the compliance of infarcted myocardium, significantly improving the post-infarctional cardiac systolic and diastolic function (Lian et al, 2002; Pijnappels et al, 2006; Mills et al, 2007). Structural and functional integration of injected cells with host myocardium is crucial to achieve a therapeutic effect.

There has been increasing concern about whether patients suffering from MI can benefit persistently from cell therapy. Not only the type and the number of transplanted cells can affect the therapeutic effect, but also the pathway and the number of transplantations. The promising therapeutic effect of MSCs relies on their convenience, in both isolation and *in vitro* expansion, as well as their ability for multipotent transdifferentiation, transfection and expression of target genes. It indicated that cell transplantation shows a dose-dependent correlation with the improvement of cardiac function. However, only a small part of transplanted cells can migrate and survive in the infarcted area and the ischemic margin of MI animal models. The efficiency of cell therapy is still challenging in its clinical application.

It had been demonstrated that an appropriate ratio of transplanted cells to host cardiomyocytes contributes to the elicitation of therapeutic effects (Chang et al, 2006). When human MSCs *in vitro* are co-cultured with neonatal cardiomyocytes at a ratio of 1:9 or 1:4, reentrant arrhythmias could be induced in 86% of the cultured system. MSCs co-cultured with neonatal cardiomyocytes at a ratio of 1:99, do not lead to the decrease in conduction velocity and reentrant arrhythmias. The number of transplanted MSCs is crucial to cardiac electrophysiological heterogenicity and arrhythmogenicity after cell transplantation. Transcoronary injection of MSCs several times to treat MI in swine models is a feasible and safe pathway for cell therapy, increasing transplantation efficiency (Poh et al, 2007). It is consistent with the results from our studies that duplicate transplantation of MSCs leads to a higher increase in cardiac function than a bolus cell injection.

We are still focusing on the optimal time points for cell transplantation in MI animal models. Consistent with the results from Lim and colleagues that a 6% increase in the cardiac function was achieved by MSCs transplantation at the early stage of acute myocardial infarction (AMI) in swine models (Lim et al, 2006), our studies showed that 2 weeks after AMI was an optimal time point to upregulate the impaired cardiac function for MSCs transplantation in rat models (Hu et al, 2007), because at the 2-week time-window inflammation was attenuated and fibrosis remained unformed (Ma et al, 2005; Bartanek et al, 2006). Optimal delivery time of bone marrow-derived stem cells (BMC) is 5 to 6 days after AMI in a REPAIR-AMI trial (Erbs et al, 2007), while no benefits can be achieved within 24 hours post-MI (Janssens et al, 2006). Another group in China, Ge JB and colleagues, had demonstrated that both 24 hours and 3-7 days post-infarction were available windows for BMC transcoronary delivery of percutaneous coronary intervention (PCI) in patients with AMI (Huang et al, 2006). Consequently, many more studies and clinical trials are needed to prove the therapeutic effects of bone marrow-derived stem cells.

4.2 Application of MSCs on Cardiomyopathy and Chronic Heart Failure

Transplantation of a bone marrow-derived stem cell, traditionally used to post-MI, is a promising therapy now being introduced to treat patients with cardiomyopathy and chronic heart failure. Results from animal studies have been carried out to ascertain the therapeutic effects. Because of diffused myocardial damage, dilated cardiomyopathy (DCM) is one of the common causes of chronic heart failure. Since evidence shows that patients with MI can benefit from MSCs transplantation due to its multipotent transdifferentiation and paracrine properties, some investigators are attempting to inject MSCs in DCM animal models.

In China, Li and colleagues (Li GC et al, 2004; Li WQ et al, 2005) had established DCM rabbit models induced by intravenous injection of doxorubicin hydrochloride for 8 weeks. Three weeks later, bone marrow-derived MSCs had been expanded *in vitro* to 1×10^6 and intramyocardially injected into the anterior wall of the left ventrium at 4 sites. Cardiac function was significantly increased after 4 weeks in rabbits with allogenic MSCs therapy compared with those of in the controls. The transplanted MSCs were found to proliferate and transdifferentiate into cardiomyocyte-like cells and endothelial cells. Neurohumoral regulation was also involved in the therapeutic effect of MSCs transplantation. A consistent result had been achieved from Zhang's studies showing that DCM rabbits could also benefit from MSCs transplantation (Zhang et al, 2007). Nagaya and colleagues (Nagaya et al, 2005) had also showed that injection of MSCs into the left ventricle of DCM rats could improve left ventricular ejection fraction (LVEF) in five weeks mediated by promoting cardiomyogensis and attenuating fibrosis. The therapeutic effects of MSCs transplantation include not only cell transdifferentiation potential, but paracrine characteristics, producing a series of pro-angiogenic, anti-apoptotic and mitogenic factors.

Chronic ischemic cardiomyopathy (ICM) is a subtype of chronic ischemic coronary disease with a high morbidity for chronic heart failure. The pathological manifestation is that of a persistent myocardial ischemia caused by diffused atherosclerosis in coronary artery, resulting in myocardial necrosis and fibrosis with an amount of hibernating and stunning cardiomyocytes. Zhu SG and collaborators had attempted bone marrow-derived cell transplantation in ICM animals (Zhu et al, 2006). They had established ICM swine models by placing an Ameroid circle at the onset of the circumflex branch of the left coronary to reduce blood flow for four weeks. Autologous bone marrow mononuclear cells (BMCs) were isolated *in vitro* and then injected intracoronary. After 4 weeks, an echocardiogram was performed to evaluate LVEF, and immunohistochemistry was used to examine capillary density. As a result, LVEF was significantly elevated and neoangioenesis was detected in ICM rats with BMCs transplantation compared to those of the controls. Their results indicated that BMC therapy might improve cardiac function of ICM patients by promoting neoangiogenesis and collateral circulation.

Diabetes mellitus (DM) is a common endocrine and metabolism disease with high morbidity and mortality. Patients with DM often suffer from some cardiovascular complications or comorbidities, including coronary heart disease (CHD), diabetic cardiomyopathy, strokes, etc., which can impair the quality of life. A successful clinical report from Brehm and Strauer showed that a DM patient complicated with extensive AMI due to complete occlusion of the left anterior descending could benefit from autologous BMCs transplantation (Brehm and Strauer, 2007). The implanted cells successfully reconstructed the damaged myocardium and blood vessels, taking on a cardiac contractile function. They assumed that myocardial repair was associated with stem cell transplantation and/or paracrine cytokine. Intracoronary stem cell transplantation may reduce the mortality of otherwise treatment-resistant cardiogenic shock. Ma and coworkers had compared the therapeutic effects of bone marrow and cord blood-derived $CD133^+$ cells in diabetic cardiomyopathy animals (Ma et al, 2006). They had isolated and prepared both kinds of stem cells, and then injected intramyocardially into NOD/SCID mice with diabetic cardiomyopathy. Both types of $CD133^+$ cells could promote noeangiogenesis and elevate survival, but only bone marrow-derived cells could improve cardiac contractility.

We tried applying bone marrow-derived MSCs to diabetic cardiomyopathy animal models (Li and Wang, 2008; Zhang et al, 2008). We established dilated cardiomyopathy models in SD rats after four months of a bolus intraperitoneal injection of streptozotocin. Rat bone marrow-derived MSCs were isolated and expanded *in vitro*. 5×10^6 of MSCs with/without anoxic preconditioning were injected intramyocardially at five sites, the right ventricular free wall, the basal and midanterior wall, the lateral wall and the posterior wall. Two weeks after transplantation, MSCs, especially anoxic preconditioned MSCs, significantly increased fractional shortening (FS)of the diabetic heart. Anoxic preconditioned MSCs increased the capillary density of diabetic myocardium and attenuated myocardial fibrosis mediated by increasing the activity of matrix metalloproteinase-2 (MMP-2) and inhibiting the transforming growth factor β_1 (TGF-β_1), respectively. Anoxic preconditioned MSCs significantly elicited anti-apoptotosis in DCM rats, possibly mediated by upregulation of Bcl-2/Bax ratio and the inhibition caspase-3 expression and activation. The results indicate that intramyocardial transplantation of MSCs have a protective effect on diabetic cardiomyopathy and anoxic preconditioning can enhance this protective effect, possibly through an anti-apoptotosis of diabetic cardiomyopathy and attenuation of cardiac remodeling.

4.3 Conclusion

In summary, bone marrow-derived stem cells are ideal candidates for cardiac celloplasty for patients with chronic heart failure and unable to receive other treatments. A multitude of animal experiments and clinical trials on stem cell transplantation are required to evaluate the therapeutic effects and their mechanisms in chronic heart failure. A cautious attitude is required concerning the results of these studies. Inconsistent results from some clinical trials have raised some questions that must be solved before clinical application. Some of these questions are as follows: What kind of patients are available for stem cell transplantation? What is the best candidate for cell therapy? When is the optimal time point for transplantation, and what is the mechanism of the therapeutic effects on cardiac function and remodeling by cell transplantation? Little evidence has been gathered on cardiomyogenesis using clinical stem cell therapy, raising more questions concerning this morbidity. How can stem cells survive and elicit biological effects in the damaged myocardium, and what percentage is necessary to generate this effect? How can we trace the biological properties of transplanted cells and evaluate their function? Is there any potential for arrhythmias or adverse effects from this cell therapy? It is critical to answer these questions before we apply stem cell transplantation to patients with heart disease. Concurrent procedures for the isolation and identification of stem cells are also crucial to objectively assess the therapeutic effect of stem cell therapy. Randomized, placebo-control clinical trials are required to further advance the application of stem cell transplantation.

References

Alvarez-Dolado M, Pardal R, Garcia-Verdugo JM, Fike JR, Lee HO, Pfeffer K, Lois C, Morrison SJ, Alvarez-Buylla A (2003) Fusion of bone-marrow-derived cells with Purkinje neurons, cardiomyocytes and hepatocytes. Nature, 425(6961):968-973

Assmus B, Schächinger V, Teupe C, Britten M, Lehmann R, Dbert N, Grnwald F, Aicher A, Urbich C, Martin H, Hoelzer D, Dimmeler S, Zeiher AM (2002) Transplantation of progenitor cells and regeneration enhancement in acute myocardial infarction. Circulation, 106(24):3009-3012

Barry FP, Murphy JM (2004) Mesenchymal stem cells: clinical application and biological properties. Int J Biochem Cell Biol, 36(4):568-584

Bartunek J, Wijns W, Heyndrickx GR, Vanderheyden M (2006) Timing of intracoronary bone-marrow-derived stem cell transplantation after ST-elevation myocardial infarction. Nat Clin Pract Cardiovasc Med, Suppl 1:S52-56

Beltrami AP, Barlucchi L, Torella D, Baker M, Limana F, Chimenti S, Kasahara H, Rota M, Musso E, Urbanek K, Leri A, Kajstura J, Nadal-Ginard B, Anversa P (2003) Adult cardiac stem cells are multipotent and support myocardial regeneration. Cell, 114(6): 763-766

Brehm M, Strauer BE (2007) Successful therapy of patients in therapy-resistant cardiogenic shock with intracoronary, autologous bone marrow stem cell transplantation. Dtsch Med Wochenschr, 132(38):1944-1948

Chang MG, Tung L, Sekar RB, Chang CY, Cysyk J, Dong PH, Marban E, Abraham MR (2006) Proarrhythmic potential of mesenchymal stem cell transplantation revealed in an *in vitro* coculture model. Circulation, 113(15):1832-1841

Chen J, Wang JA, Luo RH, Hu XY, Xie XJ, Li JH, He AN, Sun Y (2006) Effects of mesenchymal stem cells transplantation on post-infarction ventricular remodeling in rats. Chin J Emer Med, 15(4):310-314

Conget PA, Minguell JJ (2000) Adenoviral-mediated gene transfer into *ex vivo* expanded human bone marrow mesenchymal progenitor cells. Exp Hematol, 28:382-390

Ding CD, Cao KJ, Shan QJ, Zou JG, Chen ML, Jin Y (2006) Mechanism of myeloid mesenchymal stem cell transplantation in cardiac autonomic nervous function after myocardial infarction. Chin J Clin Reh, 13(10):24-28

Erbs S, Linke A, Schächinger V, Assmus B, Thiele H, Diederich KW, Hoffmann C, Dimmeler S, Tonn T, Hambrecht R, Zeiher AM, Schuler G (2007) Restoration of microvascular function in the infarct-related artery by intracoronary transplantation of bone marrow progenitor cells in patients with acute myocardial infarction: the Doppler Substudy of the Reinfusion of Enriched Progenitor Cells and Infarct Remodeling in Acute Myocardial Infarction (REPAIR-AMI) trial. Circulation, 116(4):366-374

Goldman BI, Wurzel J (2001) Evidence that human cardiac myocytes divide after myocardial infarction. N Engl J Med, 344(15):1750-1757

Hierlihy AM, Seale P, Lobe CG, Rudnicki MA, Megeney LA (2002) The post-natal heart contains a myocardial stem cell population. FEBS lett, 530(1-3):239-243

Horwitz EM, Prockop DJ, Fitzpatrick LA, Koo WW, Gordon PL, Neel M, Sussman M, Orchard P, Marx JC, Pyeritz RE, Brenner MK (1999) Transplantability and therapeutic effects of bone marrow-derived mesenchymal cells in children with osteogenesis imperfecta. Nat Med, 5(3):309-313

Hu X, Wang J, Chen J, Luo R, He A, Xie X, Li J (2007) Optimal temporal delivery of bone marrow mesenchymal stem cells in rats with myocardial infarction. Eur J Cardiothorac Surg, 31(3): 438-443

Hu X, Yu SP, Fraser J, Lu Z, Ogle ME, Wang JA, Wei L (2008) Transplantation of hypoxia preconditioned MSC improves infarcted heart function via enhanced survival of implanted cells and angiogenesis. J Thorac Cardiothorac Surg, 135(4):799-808

Huang RC, Yao K, Zhou YZ, Ge L, Qian JY, Yang J, Yang S, Niu YH, Li YL, Zhang YQ, Zhang F, Xu SK, Zhang SH, Sun AJ, Ge JB (2006) Long term follow-up on emergent intracoronary autologous bone marrow mononuclear cell transplantation for acute inferior-wall myocardial infarction. Chin J National Med, 86(16):1107-1110

Janssens S, Dubois C, Bogaert J, Theunissen K, Deroose C, Desmet W, Kalantzi M, Herbots L, Sinnaeve P, Dens J, Maertens J, Rademakers F, Dymarkowski S, Gheysens O, Van Cleemput J, Bormans G, Nuyts J, Belmans A, Mortelmans L, Boogaerts M, Van de Werf F (2006) Autologous bone marrow-derived stem-cell transfer in patients with ST-segment elevation myocardial infarction: double-blind, randomised controlled trial. Lancet, 367(9505):113-121

Kajstura J, Rota M, Whang B, Cascapera S, Hosoda T, Bearzi C, Nurzynska D, Kasahara H, Zias E, Bonaf M, Nadal-Ginard B, Torella D, Nascimbene A, Quaini F, Urbanek K, Leri A, Anversa P (2005) Bone marrow cells differentiate in cardiac cell lineages after infarction independently of cell fusion. Circ Res, 96(1):127-137

Kamihata H, Hiroaki M, Takashi N, Fujiyama S, Tsutsumi Y, Ozono R, Masaki H, Mori Y, Iba O, Tateishi E, Kosaki A, Shintani S, Murohara T, Imaizumi T, Iwasaka T (2001) Implantation of bone marrow mononuclear cells into ischemic myocardium enhances colateral perfusion and regional function via side supply of angioblasts, angiogenic ligands and cytokines. Circulation, 104 (10):1046-1052

Kawamoto A, Gwon HC, Iwaguro H, Yamaguchi JI, Uchida S, Masuda H, Silver M, Ma H, Kearney M, Isner JM, Asahara T (2001) Therapeutic potential of *ex vivo* expanded endothelial progenitor cells for myocardial ischemia. Circulation,103(5):634 -637

Li GC, Li GS, Zhang J, Li WQ, Zhou Q (2004) The empirical study of autologous bone marrow mesenchymal stem cell transplantation for dilated cardiomyopathy in rabbit. Zhonghua Xin Xue Guan Bing Za Zhi, 32(12):1095-1098

Li J, Zhang N, Wang J (2008) Improved antiapoptotic and antiremodeling potency of bone marrow mesenchymal stem cells by anoxic preconditioning in diabetic cardiomyopathy. J Endocrinol Invest, 31(2):103-110

Li WQ, Li Y, Li GC, Zhang J, Li GS (2005) Effect of autoulogous bone mesenchymal stem cell transplantation on the heart function and plasma BNP of dilated cardiomyopathy. Chin J Emerg Med, 14(7):559-562

Lian F, Zhu HS, Zheng JH, et al (2002) The research of bone marrow mesenchymal stem cell transformation into myocytes *in vitro*. Chin J Exp Surg, 19(5):454-456

Lim SY, Kim YS, Ahn Y, Jeong MH, Hong MH, Joo SY, Nam KI, Cho JG, Kang PM, Park JC (2006) The effects of mesenchymal stem cells transduced with Akt in a porcine myocardial infarction model. Cardiovasc Res, 70(3):530-542

Linke A, Muller P, Nurzynska D, Casarsa C, Torella D, Nascimbene A, Castaldo C, Cascapera S, Bohm M, Quaini F, Urbanek K, Leri A, Hintze TH, Kajstura J, Anversa P (2005) Stem cells in the dog heart are self-renewing, clonogenic, and multipotent and regenerate infarcted myocardium, improving cardiac function. Proc Natl Acad Sci USA, 102(25): 8966-8971

Liu YR, Chen JZ, Wang XX, Zhu JH, Xie XD, Sun J (2005) Changes of endothelial progenitor cells from peripheral blood in patients with coronary heart diseases. J Zhejiang Univ Sci B, 34(2):163-166

Ma J, Ge JB, Zhang SH, Wang Y, Yu Y, Sun AJ, Shi JH, Cheng LL, Shu XH, Wang KQ (2004) Improved cardiac function in the infarcted rats by intravenous transplantation of bone marrow mesenchymal stem cell. Chin J Clin Med, 11(02):151-153, 170

Ma J, Ge J, Zhang S, Sun A, Shen J, Chen L, Wang K, Zou Y (2005) Time course of myocardial stromal cell-derived factor 1 expression and beneficial effects of intravenously administered bone marrow stem cells in rats with experimental myocardial infarction. Basic Res Cardiol, 100(3):217-223

Ma N, Ladilov Y, Moebius JM, Ong L, Piechaczek C, Dvid A, Kaminski A, Choi YH, Li W, Egger D, Stamm C, Steinhoff G (2006) Intramyocardial delivery of human $CD133^+$ cells in a SCID mouse cryoinjury model: Bone marrow vs. cord blood-derived cells. Cardiovasc Res, 71(1):158-169

Makino S, Fukuda K, Miyoshi S, Konishi F, Kodama H, Pan J, Sano M, Takahashi T, Hori S, Abe H, Hata J, Umezawa A, Ogawa S (1999) Cardiomyocytes can be generated from marrow stromal cells *in vitro*. J Clin Invest, 103(5): 697-705

Matsuura K, Nagai T, Nishigaki N, Oyama T, Nishi J, Wada H, Sano M, Toko H, Akazawa H, Sato T, Nakaya H, Kasanuki H, Komuro I (2004) Adult cardiac Sca-1-positive cells differentiate into beating cardiomycytes. J Biol Chem, 279(24):11384-11391

Mills WR, Mal N, Kiedrowski MJ, Unger R, Forudi F, Popovic ZB, Penn MS, Laurita KR (2007) Stem cell therapy enhances electrical viability in myocardial infarction. J Mol Cell Cardiol, 42(2):304-314

Nagaya N, Kangawa K, Itoh T, Iwase T, Murakami S, Miyahara Y, Fujii T, Uematsu M, Ohgushi H, Yamagishi M, Tokudome T, Mori H, Miyatake K, Kitamura S (2005) Transplantation of mesenchymal stem cells improves cardiac function in a rat model of dilated cardiomyopathy. Circulation,112(8):1128-1135

Orlic D, Kajstura J, Chimenti S, Limana F, Jakoniuk I, Quaini F, Nadal-Ginard B, Bodine DM, Leri A, Anversa P (2001) Mobilized bone marrow cells repair the infarcted heart improving function and survival. Proc Natl Acad Sci USA, 98:10344-10349

Pak HN, Qayyum M, Kim DT, Hamabe A, Miyauchi Y, Lill MC, Frantzen M, Takizawa K, Chen LS, Fishbein MC, Sharifi BG, Chen PS, Makkar R (2003) Mesenchymal stem cell injection induces cardiac nerve sprouting and increased tenascin expression in a swine model of myocardial infarction. J Cardiovasc Electrophysiol, 14(8):841 -848

Partridge K, Yang X, Clarke NM, Okubo Y, Bessho K, Sebald W, Howdel SM, Shakesheff KM, Oreffo RO (2002) Adenoviral BMP-2 gene transfer in mesenchymal stem cells: *in vitro* and *in vivo* bone formation on biodegradable polymer scaffolds. Biochem Biophys Res Commun, 292(1):144-152

Pijnappels DA, Schalij MJ, van Tuyn J, Ypey DL, de Vries AA, van der Wall EE, van der Laarse A, Atsma DE (2006) Progressive increase in conduction velocity across human mesenchymal stem cells is mediated by enhanced electrical coupling. Cardiovasc Res, 72(2):282-291

Poh KK, Sperry E, Young RG, Freyman T, Barringhaus KG, Thompson CA (2007) Repeated direct endomyocardial transplantation of allogeneic mesenchymal stem cells: safety of a high dose, "off-the-shelf", cellular cardiomyoplasty strategy. Int J Cardiol, 117(3):360-364

Terada N, Hamazaki T, Oka M, Hoki M, Mastalerz DM, Nakano Y, Meyer EM, Morel L, Petersen BE, Scott EW (2002) Bone marrow cells adopt the phenotype of other cells by spontaneous cell fusion. Nature, 416(6880):542-545

Urbanek K, Quaini F, Tasca G, Torella D, Castaldo C, Nadal-Ginard B, Leri A, Kajstura J, Quaini E, Anversa P. (2003) Intense myocyte formation from cardiac stem cells in human cardiac hypertrophy. Proc Natl Acad Sci USA, 100(18):10440-10445

Urbanek K, Torella D, Sheikh F, DeAngelis A, Nurzynska D, Silvestri F, Beltrami CA, Bussani R, Beltrami AP, Quaini F, Bolli R, Leri A, Kajstura J, Anversa P (2005) Myocardial regeneration by activation of multipotent cardiac stem cells in ischemic heart failure. Proc Natl Acad Sci USA, 102(24):8692-8697

Wang JA, Li CL, Fan YQ, He H, Sun Y (2004) Allograftic bone marrow-derived mesenchymal stem cells transplanted into heart infarcted model of rabbit to renovate infarcted heart. J Zhejiang Univ Sci, 5(10):1279-1285

Wang JA, Fan YQ, Li CL, He H, Sun Y, Lv BJ (2005) Human bone marrow-derived mesenchymal stem cells transplanted into damaged rabbit heart to improve heart function. J Zhejiang Univ Sci, 6(4):242-248

Wang JA, Luo RH, Zhang X, Xie XJ, Hu XY, He AN, Chen J, Li JH (2006) Bone marrow mesenchymal stem cell transplantation combined with perindopril treatment attenuates infarction remodelling in a rat model of acute myocardial infarction. J Zhejiang Univ Sci B, 7(8): 641-647

Wang JA, He A,Hu X, Jiang Y, Sun Y, Gui C, Wang Y, Chen H (2008) Anoxic preconditioning: A way to enhance the cardio protection of mesenchymal stem cells. Int J Cardiol, (Epub ahead of print)

Wang S, Wang JA, Li J, Zhou J, Wang H (2008) Voltage-dependent potassium channels are involved in staurosporine-induced apoptosis of rat MSC. Cell Biol Int, 32(2):312-319

Zhang N, Li J, Wang J, Luo R, Jiang J (2008) Bone marrow mesenchymal stem cells induces angiogenesis and attenuates the remodeling of diabetic cardiomyopathy. Exp Clin Endocrinol, 116(2):104-111

Zhang SH, Ge JB, Qian JY, Sun AJ, Pan WM, Lin JY, Xu DL, Hu HF, Zhang F, Ma JY, Yao K, Wang QB, Liu XB, Yao RM, Shen A, Cui SJ, Wang H, Feng Q, Zou YZ, Wang KQ, Hu K (2005) Effects of bone marrow cell transplantation by coronary delivery on the different basic cardiac function degrees and its mechanisms. Chin J Clin Med, 12(6):993-995

Zhang Y, Li YL, Zhang S, Li LL, Hao DX, Gao M, Xu Y, Zhao SD (2007) Effect of autologous bone mesenchymal stem cells transplantation on the heart function of dilated cardiomyopathy. Chin J Endemiology, 26(3):273-276

Zhu SG, Xiong LH, Xie HF, Xiao SH, Hua P, Liao HY (2006) Improvement of cardiac function and promotion of angiogenesis after transplantation of autologous bone marrow mononuclear cells to chronic ischemic myocardium in swine. J SUN Yat-sen Univ (Med Sci), 27(3):293-296

5

Current Status of MSCs in Clinical Application

Jie Chen[1], **Xiaojie Xie**[2]

[1]First Affiliated Hospital, Zhejiang Tranditional Chinese Medical University, Hangzhou, China
E-mail: ktrina_cj@163.com
[2]Second Affiliated Hospital, Zhejiang University College of Medicine, Hangzhou,China
E-mail: xiaojiexie@hotmail.com

Abstract: Potential therapeutic applications of the cells require clinically compliant protocols for cell isolation and expansion. The therapeutic utility of MSCs has been evaluated and found to be useful in several pre-clinical animal models as well as in clinical trials. We review human trials studying the role of stem cell therapy in cardiomyogenesis and vasculogenesis in postinfarct myocardium, the type and number of transplanted cells, culture procedures that affect MSCs viability and quantity, time point and routes of MSCs delivery, and methods of detecting MSC engraftment. This chapter is an attempt to describe the scientific basis for MSCs therapy from the point of view of the clinician, focusing on problems that arise with beginning translation into the clinical setting.

Although modern medical technology has greatly developed, ischemic injury and heart failure are still the primary reasons for human morbility and disability all over the world. Since cardiomyocytes lack the ability to regenerate, persistent cardiac ischemia and necrosis leads to a gradual loss of myocytes, ventricular remodeling and chronic heart failure. This is the main reason for hospital admissions among the elderly.

It had been demonstrated from *in vivo* and *in vitro* studies that MSCs, which are easy to acquire and safer than other kinds of cells, can restore the injured myocardium and improve left ventricular remodeling by myogenesis and angiogenesis. The results have encouraged scientists to perform more investigations of bone marrow stem cells transplantation. The subsequent studies have been extended from a few small-scale observations to multi-centred, randomized placebo-controlled clinical trials conducted with a more objective attitude.

In recent years, an increasing amount of clinical trials relating to cell transplantation have been conducted around the world. Table 5.1 represents some famous clinical trials of cell therapy for treating patients with acute myocardial infarction (AMI) and chronic ischemic cardiomyopathy (ICM) (Roseniweig, 2006). Up to now, the REPAIR-AMT trial is the largest, clinical multi-centred and randomized, placebo-controlled study in which 204 patients with AMI (after 3 to 7 days reperfusion treatment) accepted intracoronary transplantation of autologous bone marrow mononuclear cells (BMCs) or placebo (Schächinger et al, 2006a). After treatment, left ventricular ejection fraction (LVEF) had significantly increased in four months and cardiovascular episodes including cardiac death, myocardial reinfarction, revascularization, etc., had been significantly reduced during one-year follow-up in patients with cell therapy compared to those in the control group.

Table 5.1. Comparison of clinical trials on bone marrow stem cells transplantation

Authors or Study Name	Patients Enrolled	Cell Type	Cell Number	Pathway	Time-point After AMI	Results	Side Effects	Ref.
Strauer	AMI	10 BMC	$(2.8 \pm 2.2) \times 10^7$	ICAI	5~9	Regional ventricular wall motion and blood flow improve, infarction area decreases, LVEF and LVEDV unchanged	no	(Strauer et al, 2002)
TOPCA-RE-AMI	AMI	10 NR-control 29 BMC 11 NR-control 30 CPC	$(21.3 \pm 7.5) \times 10^7$ $(1.6 \pm 1.2) \times 10^7$	ICAI	4.9 ± 1.1 4.5 ± 1.7	LVEF, LVESV, regional ventricular wall motion and myocardium energy improve, infarction area decreases, LVEDV unchanged	2 reinfarction	(Aussmus et al, 2002; Britten et al, 2003; Schächinger et al, 2004)
Chen	AMI	34 MSC	$(4.8 \sim 6.0) \times 10^{10}$	ICAI	18	LVEF,LVEDV,LVESV, regional ventricular wall motion and blood flow improve	no	(Chen et al, 2004)
Kuethe	AMI	35 R-control 5 BMC	$(3.9 \pm 2.3) \times 10^7$	ICAI	6	LVEF, regional ventricular wall motion unchanged	no	(Kuethe et al, 2004)
Katritsis	AMI	11 MSC+EPC	$(2 \sim 4) \times 10^6$	ICAI	242 ± 46	Regional ventricular wall motion and myocardium energy improve, LVEF and LV volume unchanged	no	(Katritsis et al, 2005)
Avils	AMI	13 NR-control 20 BMC	$(7.8 \pm 4.1) \times 10^7$	ICAI	14 ± 6	LVEF, LVESV, regional ventricular wall motion improve, LVEDV unchanged	1 TIA	(Avils et al, 2004)
Kang et al.	AMI	16 NR-control 7 G-CSF+CPC 3 G-CSF 1 R-control	$(150 \pm 50) \times 10^7$	ICAI	2~270	In cell transplantation group LVEF, LVESV, myocardium perfuse, coronary flow reserve improve, LVEDV unchanged	5 stent restenosis	(Kang et al, 2004)

To be continued

BOOST	AMI	30 R-control 30 NC	$(246 \pm 94) \times 10^7$	ICAI	6 ± 1	LVEF, regional ventricular wall motion (the border of the infarcts) improve, LV volume, myocardium perfuse and regional ventricular wall motion (the infarcts) unchanged	no	(Wollert et al, 2004; Meyer et al, 2006)
Janssens	AMI	30 R-control 33 BMC	$(172 \pm 72) \times 10^6$	ICAI	1	Infarction area decreases, LVEF and LV volume unchanged	no	(Janssens et al, 2006)
REPAIR-AMI	AMI	103 R-control (placebo) 101 BMC	$(23.6 \pm 17.4) \times 10^7$	ICAI	3~7	LVEF, LVESV improve, end-point incidents (death, reinfarction, readmission due to congestive heart failure) decrease, LVEDV unchanged	no	(Schächinger et al, 2006b)
ASTAMI	AMI	50 BMC 50 R-control	$(8.7 \pm 4.7) \times 10^7$	ICAI	5~8	LVEF, LVEDV, infarction area unchanged	One VT	(Lunde et al, 2005)
Lunde	AMI	50 R-control 47 BMC	68×10^6	ICAI	6	LVEF improves, LVEDV and infarction area unchanged	no	(Lunde et al, 2006)
Schächinger	AMI	103 R-control (placebo) 101 MPC	$(236 \pm 174) \times 10^6$	ICAI	4.3 ± 1.3	LVEF improves, the incidents of death, reinfarction and revascularization treatment decrease after 1 year	no	(Schächinger et al, 2006a)
Wang	AMI	11 R-control 11 MSC	$(20.2 \pm 2.91) \times 10^6$	ICAI	30~180	LVEF,LVEDV,BNP, myocardium perfuse improve	no	(Wang et al, 2005)
Tse	AMI without PCI	8 BMC	$(11.7 \pm 0.67) \times 10^6$	TEI		Symptoms relieve, regional ventricular wall motion and myocardium perfuse improve, LVEF unchanged	no	(Tse et al, 2003)
Fuchs	AMI without PCI	10 NC	$(7.8 \pm 6.6) \times 10^9$	TEI		Symptoms relieve, myocardium perfuse improve, LVEF, exercising time in treadmill test unchanged	no	(Fuchs et al, 2003)

To be continued

Perin	AMI without PCI	14 BMC 7 NR-control	$(25.5\pm6.3)\times10^6$	TEI	>90	LVEF,LVEDV, regional ventricular wall motion and myocardium perfuse improve	One SD	(Perin et al, 2003, 2004)
Kuethe	ICM	5 BMC	$(29\pm9)\times10^6$	ICAI	16±6(M)	LVEF, myocardium contraction force(the infarcts) unchanged	no	(Kuethe et al, 2005)
Strauer	ICM	18 BMC	90×10^6	ICAI	6~102(M)	Infarction area decreases, LVEF, myocardium perfuse, myocardium contraction force(the infarcts) improve	no	(Strauer et al, 2005)
Assmuss	ICM	18 NR-control 44 BMC 42 CPC	$(180\pm81)\times10^6$ $(21\pm10)\times10^6$	ICAI	3~144(M)	LVEF, stroke volume, myocardium contraction force(the infarcts), pro-ANP improve in BMC group, those unchanged in CPC group	no	(Assmus et al, 2006b)

AMI, Acute Myocardial Infarction; ICM, Ischemic Cardiomyopathy; BMC, Bone Marrow Mononuclear Cell; CPC, Circulating Progentior Cell; MSC, Mesenchymal Stem Cell; EPC, Endothelial progenitor Cell; G-CSF, Granulocyte Colony-Stimulating Factor; NC, nucleated bone marrow cell; NR-control, Non-Randomized control, R-control, Randomized control; ICAI, IntraCoronary Artery InfusionTEI,Trans-Endoscope Injection; LVEF, Left Ventricular Ejection Fraction; LVEDV, Left Ventricular End-Diastolic Volume; LVESV, Left Ventricular End-Systolic Volume; TIA, Transient Ischemic Attack; BNP, Brain Natriuretic Peptide; ANP, Atrial Natriuretic Peptide; LV, Left Ventricle; VT, Ventricular Tachycardia; SD, Sudden Death.

These findings are consistent with the preliminary results from the TOPCARE-AMI trial (Aussmus et al, 2002). When compared with controls, patients who received cell transplantation exhibited improved outcomes, including echocardiograms which demonstrated an elevation in LVEF, a decrease in left ventricular end-systolic volume (LVESV) , an increase in regional wall motion and myocardial vitality energy, and a shrinkage in the infarction area, while no significant change in left ventricular end-diastolic volume (LVEDV). Perin and colleagues (Perin et al, 2003) had performed a prospective study of cell therapy in patients with severe heart failure and without reperfusion treatment after AMI. Autologous bone marrow cells had been injected into the endocardium of the surviving myocardium by NOGA system after electrophysiologic study. The study demonstrated that myocardial blood flow was significantly increased, and regional and whole wall motion of the left ventricle was dramatically improved in patients who received cell therapy at the 4 months follow-ups.

An issue of the New England Journal of Medicine published an article comparing the therapeutic effects of the intracoronary injection of BMCs or circulation progentior cells (CPCs) in patients with AMI. It indicated that both BMCs and CPCs therapy can effectively improve the LVEF of patients with chronic ICM, which brings investigators focus on patients suffering with ICM (Assmus et al, 2006b).

A multitude of investigators and cardiologists are focusing on basic research and clinical trials of stem cell therapy to treat AMI (Ruan et al, 2005), subacute (Wang et al, 2005) and old (Wang et al, 2006; Yao et al, 2008) myocardial infarction, chronic ICM (Chen et al, 2006), chronic heart failure (Wang JA et al, 2005, 2006; Huang et al, 2006) and dilated cardiomyopathy (DCM) (Wang JA et al, 2006; Huang et al, 2006). In summary, the results are hopeful for patients afflicted with these heart diseases. Compared with the controls, cell transplantation is favorable for acute and subacute MI patients, with a limited improvement of cardiac function in patients with old myocardial infarction OMI and DCM. A meta-analysis of seven randomized, placebo-controlled clinical trials by Ge JB showed that transcoronary injection of autologous bone marrow-derived stem cells can dramatically improve post-infarcted LVEF and attenuate LVESV, but does not alleviate left ventricular remodeling (Zhang et al, 2008).

The majority of clinical trials obtain results consistent with those from animal experiments, which suggests that bone marrow cell transplantation is helpful in restoring the cardiac function in treatment of ICM. However, this issue cannot be approved due to some clinical observations listed in Table 5.1. A randomized, placebo-controlled trial, the BOOST study (Wollert et al, 2004; Meyer et al, 2006) showed that LVEF was markedly increased in patients with ST-elevated AMI after 6 months of intracoronary BMC transplantation, but demonstrated no statistical difference in an 18-month follow-up. The results from Janssens studies (Janssens et al, 2006) showed intracoronary BMC injection does not attenuate LVEF, but does shrink the infarcted area in ST-elevated AMI patients. A recent report of the ASTAMI studies demonstrates that it safe for intracoronary BMC transplantation in MI patients for a short term, but there is no increase in LVEF detected by cardiac MRI and PET examinations (Lunde, 2005, 2006).

With regards to the clinical trials discussed above, it becomes apparent that procedures of cell transplantation should be standardized, making different study results comparable. The inconsistency among the conclusions is also affected by the complexity of clinical observations. The possible reasons for the discrepancy regarding the cardiac function in stem cell therapy might include the following.

5.1 The Type and Number of Transplanted Cells

Bone marrow-derived cells are one of the most widely used cell categories in clinical trials, including multiple undifferentiated progenitor cells, mesenchymal stem cells (MSCs), hemopoietic stem cells (HSCs) and endothelial progenitor cells (EPCs). Compared with embryonic stem cells (ESCs), cord blood-derived stem cell and skeletal myoblast, MSCs have a series of advantages, such as plenty of resources, no ethical dispute, and apparent safety in clinical application. Bone marrow mononuclear cells (BMCs) are available in a variety of clinical studies, such as TOPARE-AMI, BOOST and REPAIRING-AMI. It is difficult to compare the therapeutic effects of different cell types in these clinical trials because the evidence cannnot clarify which one is the best candidate. The biology of adult cardiac stem cells begs the question of whether function can be restored. Bone marrow-derived MSCs are undifferentiated cells which do not express CD34 and CD133. They have been demonstrated to transdifferentiate into cardiomyocytes *in vivo* and *in vitro*. The application of MSCs to treat MI appears to restore cardiac function and attenuate left ventricular remodeling, while the mechanisms are still unclarified. As for regenerative medicine, cell therapy is still a promising method of heart function restoration, although it requires further investigation. In addition, MSCs may be the best candidate for allogenetic transplantation due to their low immunogenicity.

It's indicated that MSCs can restore cardiac function mediated by cardiomyogenesis, neoangiogenesis and paracrine mechanisms. The execution of these effects depends on a certain number of stem cells surviving in the infarcted myocardium. Whatever pathways are available to cell transplantation (intravenous, intramyocardial, transcoronary or endomyocardial), stem cells homing into the ischemic myocardium and executing their protective effects is crucial to cell therapy. Since evidence has shown that only 1.3% to 2.6% of transplanted bone marrow cells can survive in the infarcted myocardium, it's likewise critical to maintain transplanted cells surviving in the cardiac microenvironment. Engrafted cells cannot reach to the infarcted margin via the common pathway of transplantation; therefore the efficacy is "bottlenecked" as regards its clinical application. In the majority of clinical trials, the amount of stem cells injected was $10^6 - 10^9$. Our studies show that $(20.2 \pm 2.91) \times 10^6$ of MSCs exhibits a therapeutic effect on the cardiac function in post-MI patients. There are no reports of the correlation between cell numbers and their effect on clinical prognosis. Ge JB and colleagues had claimed that repeated transplantation led to marked improvement in the cardiac function, rather than a bolus injection. It is still not clear whether an increased number of transplanted cells results in better therapeutic effects without microthrombosis. The type and number of candidate cells for transplantation may contribute to the clinical therapeutic effects.

5.2 Cell Preparation

As mentioned above, while the therapeutic effects of stem cell therapy discovered in the REPAIR-AMI trial are inspiring, they are inopposition to the result from the ASTAMI trial. Seeger and collaborators had compared the difference between transplanted cells in these two trials (Seeger et al, 2007). For the REPAIR-AMI trial, BMCs were aspirated from bone marrow separated by gradient centrifugation onto Ficoll and incubated overnight in X-vivo medium supplemented with 20% autologous serum at room temperature. In the ASTAMI trial, BMCs were overlaid and and separated by different densities of lympocyte-isolating solution, and then incubated with saline supplemented by 20% serum containing heparin. More MSCs expressing $CD45^+/CD34^+$ and $CD45^+/CD133^+$ can be isolated and purfied by Ficoll than other substrates. The cells had the typical characteristics of a stem cell, such as clone-forming and migration in the presence of chemokines, SDF-1. In hind limb ischemia mice models, MSCs isolated by Ficoll and transplanted showed markedly increased blood flow in the hind limbs, compared with those acquired by lymphocyte-isolating solution. The discrepancies in preparation procedures could influence the phenotype and function of cells, and thus their therapeutic effects after transplantation. Modification and standardization of cell preparation to ensure the proper number and effective biological properties is attracting investigators' attention.

5.3 The Time Point and Pathway of Cell Transplantation

The dynamic balance of cardiac injury and repair is a complicated pathological process, involving cell ischemia, apoptosis and necrosis, cytokines accumulation and scar formation. Myocardial synthesis and repair is overwhelming when damage is not fatal. The cardiac microenvironment is crucial to the migration, adhesion, retention, survival and differentiation of the transplanted cells. It's unclear when the optimal time window of cell transplantation is present to achieve the best therapeutic effect. In most studies, the time point of cell transplantation has ranged from one day to several months after MI. We had established AMI models in SD rats by ligration of left anterior descending and intramyocardially injected allogenic bone marrow-derived MSCs (Hu et al, 2007). Exogenous cells survived longer in the cardiac microenvironment at one week than at one hour or two weeks after AMI. Ge JB and his colleagues had enrolled 104 patients with ST-elevated AMI and randomly divided them into four groups, BMCs or placebo were injected into the culprit artery either immediately, 3～7 days or 7～30 days after PCI. Their results showed that in a 12-month follow-up LVEF was markedly elevated, and left ventricular end-systolic dimension (LVESDs) and infarction area decreased in patients treated with BMCs post-PCI immediately or 3～7 days after PCI than those treated with BMCs 7～30 days after PCI. There was no significance in the therapeutic effects between patients treated with BMCs post-PCI immediately and 3～7 days after PCI (Zhao et al, 2005). The results indicated that immediately may be the best time-point of cell transplantation for treating patients with AMI, with a short time for hospitalization, low expenses and great therapeutic effects. A recent report indicated that administration of intracoronary bone marrow monoclear cells on chronic MI can improve diastolic function (Yao et al, 2008).

Presently, the common pathways for cell transplantation in clinical trials include transplantation via intracoronary, intravenous, sub-endocardial by NOGA system, epicardium injection during surgery or under thoracoscope, etc. The purpose of having different options for cell therapy is to make it more convenient, effective and safe for patients treated with stem cells.

5.4 Others

The criteria for patients enrolled into the trials are key to the conclusions of the studies. The accumulation of study cases contributes to objective and accurate conclusions. Precise examinations are available to evaluate cardiac function and make persuasive arguments. Long-term follow-up is crucial to assess a new therapy. The results of the BOOST trial displayed that a 6 to 8 months follow-up was ideal.

In addition to the effectiveness of a new therapy, safety is also a critical issue to be addressed. Investigators are focusing on some adverse effects after cell transplantation, such as restenosis, reinfarction, and proarrhythmias. Kang and colleagues had intracoronary injection of bone marrow cells combined with granulocyte colony-stimulating factor (G-CSF) in AMI patients, who accepted PCI and bare stenting in the culprit coronary. Five patients treated with G-CSF (5/7) had restenosis occur at the stents. Results from Mansours' studies showed that intracoronary injection of $CD133^+$ bone marrow cells led to significant cell proliferation in stents and restenosis in the distal branches of the infarction-related artery uncovered by the stent , and thus cut off the blood flow. Evidence from these two trials dims the hopes of intracoronary cell therapy somewhat. However, Assmus (Assmus et al, 2006a) deemed that neither restenosis in stents nor revascularization occurred during transcoronary transplantation of bone marrow stem cells. In MAGIC-Cell studies, 154 AMI patients had been injected intracoronarily with CPCs combined with G-CSF. The results were inconsistent in a 2-year follow-up that this combination therapy can inhibit cell proliferation, promote endothelium healing and prevent thrombosis in eluting stents. In China, Li and Liu had demonstrated that bone marrow progenitor cells mobilized by G-CSF were homing in on the infarcted myocardium, improving global left ventricular function and attenuating ventricular remodeling with no obvious adverse effects at the 6-month follow-up, which indicated a safe and feasible treatment for patients with AMI. In fact this is a larger scale clinical test which researches using multi-regression analysis, and also considers that diabetes is a dependent dangerous element for stent restenosis, other than in cell treatment by multi-regression analysis. Actually, multi-regression analysis of a series of clinical trials implied that diabetes mellitus (DM) is an independent risk factor for restenosis, but not cell therapy.

Aggravation of coronary restenosis after intracoronary cell therapy was observed by Kang and Mansour to be attributable to proinflammatory effects of G-CSF and the preparation process of bone marrow cells. When drug-eluting stents (DES) were used instead of bare stents, Kang and colleagues found that the combination therapy of G-CSF and cell transplantation did not lead to stent restenosis, but by contrast improved LVEF (Kang et al, 2004). Results from MAGIC Study further proved that stem cell therapy does not increase the occurence of stent restenosis based on DES application. It more likely that the anti-inflammation effects of DES could balance the pro-inflammation caused by G-CSF. Therefore, pro-atherosclerosis caused by intracoronary cell transplantation is based on the procedures of cell transplantation rather than the transplanted cell itself.

The safety of intracoronary transplantation of antologous bone marrow stem cells is further proved by the SEACOAST trial (from TCT 2007 report). Nine chronic ICM patients were enrolled in the study and an intracoronary injection of different numbers of $CD133^+$ cells were used. No adverse effects were reported in a 6-month follow-up, including secondary MI, arrhythmias, elevation of cardiac enzymes, and myocardial perfusion was dramatically improved in 6 patients. Meta-analysis of five randomized, placebo-controlled studies by Ge JB indicated that it is safe to perform intracoronary transplantaion of bone marrow cells to treat patients with AMI. MSC transplantation at 4~7 days after PCI is much safer than 24 hours post-PCI (Zhang et al, 2008).

The majority of clinical trials have implied that cell transplantation does not cause malignant arrhythmias as expected. It might be associated with the expression of Connexin 43 on bone marrow stem cells, which form an electrical coupling with cardiomyocytes rather than skeletal myoblasts. There are no reports of any malignant tumors due to stem cell hyperplasia. Based on these points, bone marrow stem cell transplantation may be easier to be clinially adopted.

5.5 Conclusion

In summary, evidences from multitudes of clinical trials indicate that bone marrow cells transplantation is a safe procedure, and appears to be effective in patients with ICM (Table 5.1). Final conclusions are still unclarified, and the mechanisms involved are still being disputed. The discrepancies of paracrine effects or transdifferentiation characteristics is coexistent. Clinical trials should be based on the results and objective analysis of multiple experiments using animal models.

We are expecting a new future for gene therapy and cell engineering.

References

Assmus B, Walter DH, Lehmann R, Honold J, Martin H, Dimmeler S, Zeiher AM, Schächinger V (2006a) Intracoronary infusion of progenitor cells is not associated with aggravated restenosis development or atherosclerotic disease progression in patients with acute myocardial infarction. Eur Heart J, 27(23):2989-2995

Assmus B, Honold J, Schächinger V, Britten MB, Fischer-Rasokat U, Lehmann R, Teupc C, Pistorius K, Martin H, D. Abolmaali N, Tonn T, Dimmeler S, Zeiher AM (2006b) Transcoronary transplantation of progenitor cells after myocardial infarction. N Engl J Med, 355(12):1222-1232

Aussmus B, Schächinger V, Teupe C, Britten M, Lehmann R, Dbert N, Grnwald F, Aicher A, Urbich C, Martin H, Hoelzer D, Dimmeler S, Zeiher AM (2002) Transplantation of progenitor cells and regeneration enhancement in acute myocardial infarction (TOPCARE-AMI). Circulation, 106(24):3009-3017

Avils FF, San Romn JA, Garca Frade J, Valds M, Snchez A, de la Fuente L, Pearrubia MJ, Fernndez ME, Tejedor P, Durn JM, Hernndez C, Sanz R, Garca Sancho J (2004) Intracoronary stem cell transplantation in acute myocardial infarction. Rev Esp Cardiol, 57(3):201-208

Britten MB, Abolmaali ND, Assmus B, Lehmann R, Honold J, Schmitt J, Vogl TJ, Martin H, Schächinger V, Dimmeler S, Zeiher AM (2003) Infarct remodeling after intracoronary progenitor cell treatment in patients with acute myocardial infarction (TOPCARE-AMI): mechanistic insights from serial contrast-enhanced magnetic resonance imaging. Circulation, 108(18):2212-2218

Chen SL, Fang WW, Ye F, Liu YH, Qian J, Shan SJ, Zhang JJ, Chunhua RZ, Liao LM, Lin S, Sun JP (2004) Effect on left ventricular function of intracoronary transplantation of autologous bone marrow mesenchymal stem cell in patients with acute myocardial infarction. Am J Cardiol, 94(1):92-95

Chen S, Liu Z, Tian N, Zhang J, Yei F, Duan B, Zhu Z, Lin S, Kwan TW (2006) Intracoronary transplantation of autologous bone marrow mesenchymal stem cells for ischemic cardiomyopathy due to isolated chronic occluded left anterior descending artery. J Invasive Cardiol, 18(11):552-556

Fuchs S, Satler LF, Kornowski R, Okubagzi P, Weisz G, Baffour R, Waksman R, Weissman NJ, Cerqueira M, Leon MB, Epstein SE (2003) Catheter-based autologous bone marrow myocardial injection in no-option patients with advanced coronary artery disease: a feasibility study. J Am Coll Cardiol, 41(10):1721-1724

Hu XY, Wang JA, Chen J, Luo RH, He AN, Xie XJ, Li JH, Zhang X, Min JY (2007) Optimal temporal delivery of bone marrow mesenchymal stem cells in rats with myocardial infarction. Eur J Cardiothorac Surg, 31(3):438-443

Huang RC, Yao K, Li YL, Zhang YQ, Xu SK, Shi HY, Pan CZ, Yang S, Zhang SH, Ge L, Niu YH, Zhang F, Qian JY, Zou YZ, Ge JB (2006) Transplantation of autologous bone marrow mononuclear cells on patients with idiopathic dilated cardiomyopathy: early results on effect and security. Chin J Cardiovasc, 34(2):111-113

Janssens S, Dubois C, Bogaert J, Theunissen K, Deroose C, Desmet W, Kalantzi M, Herbots L, Sinnaeve P, Dens J, Maertens J, Rademakers F, Dymarkowski S, Gheysens O, Van Cleemput J, Bormans G, Nuyts J, Belmans A, Mortelmans L, Boogaerts M, Van de Werf F (2006) Autologous bone marrow-derived stem-cell transfer in patients with ST-segment elevation myocardial infarctin: double-blind, randomized controlled trial. Lancet, 367(9505):113-121

Kang HJ, Kim HS, Zhang SY, Park KW, Cho HJ, Koo BK, Kim YJ, Soo Lee D, Sohn DW, Han KS, Oh BH, Lee MM, Park YB (2004) Effects of intracoronary infusion of peripheral blood stem-cells mobilised with granulocyte-colony stimulating factor on left ventricular systolic function and restenosis after coronary stenting in myocardial infarction: the MAGIC cell randomised clinical trial. Lancet, 363(9411):751-756

Katritsis DG, Sotiropoulou PA, Karvouni E, Karabinos I, Korovesis S, Perez SA, Voridis EM, Papamichail M (2005) Transcoronary transplantation of autologous mesenchymal stem cells and endothelial progenitors into infarcted human myocardium. Catheter Cardiovasc Interv, 65(3):321-329

Kuethe F, Richartz BM, Sayer HG, Kasper C, Werner GS, Hffken K, Figulla HR (2004) Lack of regeneration of myocardium by autologous intracoronary mononuclear bone marrow cell transplantation in humans with large anterior myocardial infarctions. Int J Cardiol, 97(1):123-127

Kuethe F, Richartz BM, Kasper C, Sayer HG, Hoeffken K, Werner GS, Figulla HR (2005) Autologous intracoronary mononuclear bone marrow cell transplantation in chronic ischemic cardiomyopathy in humans. Int J Cardiol, 100(3):485-491

Lunde K, Solheim S, Aakhus S, Arnesen H, Abdelnoor M, Egeland T, Endresen K, Ilebekk A, Mangschau AG. Fjeld J, Smith HJ, Taraldsrud E, Groaard H K, Bjonerheim R, Brekke M, Mller C, Hopp E, Ragnarsson A, Brinchmann JE, Forfang K (2005) Autologous stem cell transplantation in acute myocardial infarction: The ASTAMI randomized controlled trial. Intracoronary transplantation of autologous mononuclear bone marrow cells, study design and safety aspects. Scand Cardiovasc J, 39(3):150-158

Lunde K, Solheim S, Aakhus S, Arnesen H, Abdelnoor M, Egeland T, Endresen K, Ilebekk A, Mangschau A, Fjeld JG, Smith HJ, Taraldsrud E, Grgaard HK, Bjrnerheim R, Brekke M, Mller C, Hopp E, Ragnarsson A, Brinchmann JE,

Forfang K (2006) Intracoronary injection of mononuclear bone marrow cells in acute myocardial infarction. N Engl J Med, 355(12):1199-1209

Meyer GP, Wollert KC, Lotz J, Steffens J, Lippolt P, Fichtner S, Hecker H, Schaefer A, Arseniev L, Hertenstein B, Ganser A, Drexler H (2006) Intracoronary bone marrow cell transfer after myocardial infarction: eighteen months?follow-up data from the randomized, controlled BOOST trial. Circulation, 113(10):1287-1294

Perin EC, Dohmann HF, Borojevic R, Silva SA, Sousa AL, Mesquita CT, Rossi MI, Carvalho AC, Dutra HS, Dohmann HJ, Silva GV, Belm L, Vivacqua R, Rangel FO, Esporcatte R, Geng YJ, Vaughn WK, Assad JA, Mesquita ET, Willerson JT (2003) Transendocardial, autologous bone marrow cell transplantation for severe, chronic ischemic heart failure. Circulation,107(18):2294-2302

Perin EC, Dohmann HF, Borojevic R, Silva SA, Sousa AL, Silva GV, Mesquita CT, Belm L, Vaughn WK, Rangel FO, Assad JA, Carvalho AC, Branco RV, Rossi MI, Dohmann HJ, Willerson JT (2004) Improved exercise capacity and ischemia 6 and 12 months after transendocardial injection of autologous bone marrow mononuclear cells for ischemic cardiomyopathy. Circulation, 110(11 Suppl 1):II213-218

Rosenzweig A (2006) Cardiac cell therapy-mixed results from mixed cells. N Engl J Med, 355(12):1274-1277

Ruan W, Pan CZ, Huang GQ, Li YL, Ge JB, Shu XH (2005) Assessment of left ventricular segmental function after autologous bone marrow stem cells transplantation in patients with acute myocardial infarction by tissue tracking and strain imaging. Chin Med J (Engl), 118(14):1175-1181

Schächinger V, Assmus B, Britten MB, Honold J, Lehmann R, Teupe C, Abolmaali ND, Vogl TJ, Hofmann WK, Martin H, Dimmeler S, Zeiher AM (2004) Transplantation of progenitor cells and regeneration enhancement in acute myocardial infarction: final one-year results of the TOPCARE-AMI Trial. J Am Coll Cardiol, 44(8):1690-1699

Schächinger V, Erbs S, Elsasser A, Haberbosch W, Hambrecht R, Holschermann H, Yu J, Corti R, Mathey DG, Hamm CW, Suselbeck T, Assmus B, Tonn T, Dimmeler S, Zeiher AM (2006a) Improved clinical outcome after intracoromary administration of bone marrow derived progenitor cells in acute myocardial infarction: final 1-year results of the REPAIR-AMI trial. Eur Heart J, 27(23):2775-2783

Schächinger V, Erbs S, Elssser A, Haberbosch W, Hambrecht R, Hlschermann H, Yu J, Corti R, Mathey DG, Hamm CW, Sselbeck T, Assmus B, Tonn T, Dimmeler S, Zeiher AM. REPAIR-AMI Investigators (2006b) Intracoronary bone marrow-derived progenitor cells in acute myocardial infarction. N Engl J Med, 355(12):1210-1221

Seeger FH, Tonn T, Krzossok N, Zeiher AM, Dimmeler S (2007) Cell isolation procedures matter: a comparison of different isolation protocols of bone marrow mononuclear cells used for cell therapy in patients with acute myocardial infarction. Eur Heart J, 28(6):766-772

Strauer BE, Brehm M, Zeus T, Kstering M, Hernandez A, Sorg RV, Kgler G, Wernet P (2002) Repair of infarcted myocardium by autologous intracoronary mononuclear bone marrow cell transplantation in humans. Circulation, 106(15):1913-1918

Strauer BE, Brehm M, Zeus T, Bartsch T, Schannwell C, Antke C, Sorg RV, Kgler G, Wernet P, Mller HW, Kstering M (2005) Regeneration of human infarcted heart muscle by intracoronary autologous bone marrow cell transplantation in chronic coronary artery disease: the IACT Study. J Am Coll Cardiol, 46(9):1651-1658

Tse HF, Kwong YL, Chan JK, Lo G, Ho CL, Lau CP (2003) Angiogenesis in ischaemic myocardium by intramyocardial autologous bone marrow mononuclear cell implantation. Lancet, 361(9351):47-49

Wang JA, Xie XJ, Sun Y, He H, Jiang CY, Zhou BQ, Luo RH, Dong L (2005) Autologous mesenchymal stem cells transplantation in patients with post-myocardial infarction and cardiac dysfunction. Chin J Emerg Med, 14(12):996-999

Wang JA, Xie XJ, He H, Sun Y, Jiang J, Luo RH, Fan YQ, Dong L (2006) A prospective, randomized, controlled trial of autologous mesenchymal stem cells transplantation for dilated cardiomyopathy. Zhonghua Xin Xue Guan Bing Za Zhi, 34(2):107-110

Wang WM, Sun NL, Liu J, Zhang P, Liu KY, Wang Q, Yang SN, Wang SQ, Zang Y, Guo JH (2006) Effects of intracoronary autologous bone marrow mononuclear cells transplantation in patients with anterior myocardial infarction. Zhonghua Xin Xue Guan Bing Za Zhi, 34(2):103-106

Wollert KC, Meyer GP, Lotz J, Ringes-Lichtenberg S, Lippolt P, Breidenbach C, Fichtner S, Korte T, Hornig B, Messinger D, Arseniev L, Hertenstein B, Ganser A, Drexler H (2004) Intracoronary autologous bone-marrow cell transfer after myocardial infarction: the BOOST randomized controlled clinical trial. Lancet, 364(9429):141-148

Yao K, Huang R, Qian J, Cui J, Ge L, Li Y, Zhang F, Shi H, Huang D, Zhang S, Sun A, Zou Y, Ge J (2008) Administration of intracoronary bone marrow mononuclear cells on chronic myocardial infarction improues diastolic function. Heart, 94(9):1147-1153

Zhang SN, Sun AJ, Ge JB, Yao K, Huang ZY, Wang KQ, Zou YZ (2008) Intracoronary autologous bone marrow stem cells transfer for patients with acute myocardial infarction: A meta-analysis of randomised controlled trials. Jul 19 [Epub ahead of print]

Zhao Y, GE J, Zhang S, Qian J, Sun A, Wang K, Shi J, Hu K, Zou Y (2005) Optimal time for bone marrow cells transplantation to maximize heart function after myocardial infarction. Zhongguo Lin Chuang Yi Xue, 12(2):192-195

6

MSCs as a Vector of Gene Engineering

Tielong Chen[1]**, Xiaojie Xie**[2]

[1]Hangzhou Hospital of Tranditional Chinese Medicine,
Hangzhou,China
E-mail: ctlppp@sohu.com
[2]Second Affiliated Hospital, Zhejiang University College of Medicine,
Hangzhou, China
E-mail: xiaojiexie@hotmail.com

Abstract: Introduction of transgene of interest into autologous stem cell types poses an attractive cell-based delivery strategy. Gene delivery to MSCs has been proposed as a mechanism to promote the augmentation of tissue-engineered replacement systems. MSCs are attractive targets for gene delivery systems, because they can differentiate, in response to various molecular signals, into many types of committed cells. MSCs divide rapidly and are readily transducible with integrating vectors and maintain transgene expression *in vitro* and *in vivo* without affecting multipotentiality. The unique biology of MSCs predetermines them to become valuable cytoreagents for gene therapy approaches in future. This chapter briefly describes the application of MSCs in genetic engineering according to the category of vectors and desired nucleic acid.

Genetically modified mesenchymal stem cells (MSCs) are a valuable tool for the novel treatment of human diseases, especially in the heart. MSCs are pluripotent cells that are considered an important resource for human cell-based therapies. Gene transference into MSCs with subsequent expression has become a valuable tool for physiological studies, functional genomics and gene therapy. Furthermore, ectopic expression of signaling molecules and transcription factors is useful for manipulating the differentiation, immigration and apoptosis of cells. It is a key factor in choosing suitable recipient cells for successful gene therapy. Recipient cells for gene therapy should be easily acquired and cultured and have a long lifespan. Recently, on account of these requirements, scientists have begun to pay more attention to stem cells, such as embryonic stem cell (ESC), hematopoietic stem cell (HSC) and MSC,etc. MSCs have some advantages over other kinds of stem cells; they are readily obtained from bone marrow, are easily isolated and expanded *ex vivio*, they have low immunogenicity with regards to engraft rejection, and their use is unrestricted by ethics. It has also demonstrated from a series of animal studies that MSCs can be regarded as ideal candidates for target gene transfection and expression.

The common vectors of gene engineering include viral vectors and nonviral vectors, such as retrovirus, adenovirus, lentivirus, liposomes and plasmids, etc. The caveat concerning the combination of gene and cell therapy is whether vectors can confer transgenic expression to the host cells without any cytotoxicity. Generally, MSCs are easily transfected and carry exogenous genes with a relatively high expression. McMahon and colleagues had compared the efficiency of a broad range of both viral and nonviral vectors at delivering green fluorescent protein (GFP) reporter gene into rat MSCs as well as determining the effect of these procedures on cell survival (McMahon et al, 2006). Lentivirus proved to be most effective with transfection efficiencies of up to 95%, and concurrent with low cytotoxicity. Adenovirus also proved effective, but a significant increase in cell death was seen with increasing viral titration. Rat MSCs remained refractory to transduction by all adeno-associated virus (AAV) serotypes, in contrast to rabbit MSCs tested at the same time. Approximately 93% of MSCs transfected by AAV could express target genes and the related proteins. Retrovirus is able to transfect MSCs quite easily, but the efficiency is decreased to 50%∼80%. Lipofection of plasmid DNA gave moderate transduction levels but was also accompanied by cell death. Electroporative gene transfer proved ineffective at the parameters tested and resulted in high cell death. Cationic lipid-mediated transduction had been demonstrated to be highly ineffective as well as causing serious cytotoxicity to MSCs. High and moderate levels of cell transfection using lentivirus vectors did not affect the ability of the cells to differentiate down the adipogenic pathway. In summary, lentivirus might be the best vector for transfection in MSCs.

According to different target genes and their vectors, we will briefly introduce the application of MSCs in genetic engineering.

6.1 Adenoviruses and Angiogenesis-related Genes

Adenovirus is a type of non-enveloped viruses containing a linear double stranded DNA genome. There are 42 serotypes of adenovirus known to infect humans and most of the adenoviral vectors used for gene therapy are based on serotype 2 and 5. Adenovirus is a popular vector for gene therapy because of its suberb transduction efficiency and high levels of transgene expression both in mitogenic or non-mitogenic cells. Adenovirus, as a safe vector, has the following characteristics as follows. It does not lead to any diseases or cancer, but may cause slight symptoms. Adenovirus will transfect a broad range of cells, both mitogenic and non-mitogenic. Usually the target gene is up to 4.7~4.9 kbp and even 8.3 kbp for a new subtype of adenovirus vector, which could not be integrated into the host chromosome and expressed persistently (around 1~6 weeks). Advenovirus has a stable structure and immunogenicity, once recombined with a host genome or other virus. The reconstruction of the advenovirus vector involves inserting the target gene into a small shuttle plasmid, and thereby the cassette is integrated into the adenovirus via the plasmid.

Bone marrow-derived MSCs can be effectively transfected by advenovirus with a minimal effect on cell survival. According to Li HL and colleagues' studies, recombinant advenovirus vector carrying a target gene of brain-derived neurotrophic factor (BDNF) can effectively transfect bone marrow-derived MSCs with an efficiency of 36% (Li et al, 2003). Guo and colleagues had successfully transfected bone marrow MSCs with recombinant advenvirus vector carrying the *SERCA-2a* gene. No obvious cytotoxicity was observed, and transfection efficiency was up to 83.8% in MSCs by flow cytometry analysis in 7 days. Expression of *SERCA-2a* in transcriptional (mRNA) and translational (protein) levels had also been detected (Guo and Li, 2003).

Vascular endothelial growth factor (VEGF) plays an important role in promoting neoangiogenesis. The human *VEGF165* gene can be successfully transfected into the cultured rat MSCs using an adenoviral vector (Matsumoto et al, 2005). Six millions MSCs co-transfected with *VEGF* and *LacZ* gene (as a reporter gene) were injected into a syngeneic rat AMI heart one hour after left coronary artery ligation in VEGF group. At 28 days after AMI, infarct size, left ventricular dimensions, left ventricular ejection fraction (LVEF), E/A ratio and capillary density of the infarcted region were dramatically improved in rats of VEGF group, compared with those of the controls. Consistent results have been obtained from a series of animal studies (Gao et al, 2007; Zhou et al 2006; Yang et al, 2007; Guan et al, 2006). Transplantation of *VEGF* gene-transfected MSCs delivers a major improvement and better restoration of the cardiac function than either cell or gene therapy alone.

Angiopoietin-I (AngI) has been shown to not only be specific and critical for angiogenesis, but to have a protective effect on cardiomyocytes *in vitro*. Human AngI (*hAngI*) gene could be transfected into cultured rat MSCs mediated by an adenoviral vector. Five million *hAngI*-transfected MSCs (*AngI*-MSC) or green fluorescent protein transfected MSCs (*GFP*-MSC) were injected intramyocardialy into inbred Lewis rat hearts immediately after experimental myocardial infarction. Ventricular remodeling was attenuated and cardiac function was improved in rats of both the (*AngI*-MSC) and *GFP*-MSC groups. However, in contrast to those of *GFP*-MSC group, rats of *AngI*-MSC group presented enhanced angiogenesis and arteriogenesis (by 11%~35%), while the infarction area was reduced by 30% and the left ventricular wall was 46% thicker (Sun et al, 2007).

6.2 Adeno-associated Virus (AAV) and Anti-inflammation Related Genes

Adeno-associated virus (AAV) is a dependent parvovirus with a 4,679 base single-stranded linear genome that contains two open reading frames, namely Rep and Cap. Rep is a nonstructural protein involved in rescue and replication of the virus, while Cap forms an icosahederal capsid within which the replicated genome is packaged. There are three different promoters in the AAV genome,which are p5, p19, and p40. In addition to the Rep and Cap genes, the AAV genome typically contains a transgene expression cassette flanked by the virally inert terminal repeats (ITRs). The ITRs are the sole elements required for rescue, replication, packaging and integration of AAV, which are rich in GC bases and form a hairpin structure with three complementary domains that form a double-stranded structure. The package system consists of recombination vector, helper vector, helper virus and incasing cells. Since AAV is a nonpathogenic virus as well as replication-incompetent, it has innate "safety" features. Although AAV can transfect a broad range of host cells, including mitogenic and non-mitogenic, only less than 5 kbp target genes can be packaged in AAV with a limited ability of transfection. Helper viruses such as adenovirus are required for viral genome replication and thus synthesizing AVV proteins. There are no reports of wild type AAV associated with human diseases. All types of AAV including scAAVs, $scAAV_2$ and $scAAV_5$ can transfect MSCs in a safe and effective manner, with 60%~70% efficiency for $scAAV_2$ and a 3-month expression of target gene after transfection.

Bao and colleagues had transfected rat bone marrow-derived MSCs with recombinant AAV to carry a tumor necrosis factor receptor *(TNFR)* gene, and then intramyocardialy injected rAAV-*TNFR* MSCs into the infarcted myocardium (Bao et al, 2007). Consequently, compared with those of cell therapy alone, *TNFR*-transfected MSCs had a significantly improved left ventricular function in AMI animals by the mechanisms of anti-apoptosis and anti-inflammation. Also, MSCs-*TNFR* transplantation attenuated the synthesis of pro-inflammatory cytokines in the cardiac microenvironment, such as TNF-alpha, interleukin -1 beta (IL-1β) and IL-6.

6.3 Retrovirus and Anti-apoptosis Related Genes

Recombinant retroviruses are one of the most commonly used vectors for gene therapy. A retroviral vector is a single-stranded RNA virus and consists of two copies of viral RNA, each containing complete genomic informations acquired for virus replication. The retrovirus has a lipid envelope, which can interact with cell membrane receptors or be embedded to enter host cells. A recombinant retrovirus has a broad range of host cells (mitogenic cells only) and a great transfection efficiency without serious cytotoxicity. Retrovirus vectors could transfer their genomic information to the daughter cells through binding to the host genome. It is possible to produce a wild type recombinant retrovirus possessing powerful replication; therefore the vectors and packing cells are required to be reconstructed in case of contamination.

Nonassociated sequences might be integrated into host cells and lead to inaccuracy of genomic recombination. Compared to an advenovirus, a retrovirus can hold exogenous genes up to 7 kbp with a low viral titration.

Bone marrow-derived MSCs can be easily transfected by retrovirus vectors with an effeciency of 50%~80%. Liu GB and colleagues had transfected rat MSCs with recombinant retrovirus and claimed that the percentage of retrovirus-transfected cells reporting enhanced GFP (EGFP) was around 21%, at a transfection interval of more than 20 days, while merely 3% of liposome-transfected MSCs were reported with EGFP (Zheng et al, 2005).

An anti-apoptotic protein 26-kDa *Bcl-2* belongs to the proteins of the *Bcl-2* family, which serves as a critical regulator involved in apoptosis signaling, alleviating cell death. Rat MSCs had been transfected to overexpress the *Bcl-2* gene, which could reduce MSCs apoptosis by 32% and enhance VEGF secretion by more than 60% under hypoxic conditions. Capillary density in the infarct border zone was 15% higher in *Bcl-2*-MSCs transplanted animals than those of vector-MSCs treated animals. Furthermore, *Bcl-2*-MSCs transplanted animals had a 17% smaller infarct size than vector-MSCs treated animals and exhibited marked functional restoration (Li et al, 2007). The survival of *Bcl-2*-MSCs was 1.2 to 2.2 folders higher than vector-MSCs. Transplantation of anti-apoptotic gene-modified MSCs may have a crucial role for mediating substantial functional restoration after acute myocardial infarction (AMI).

Akt, a serine threonine kinase, is a powerful survival signal in many systems. Mangi and colleagues had genetically engineered rat MSCs using *ex vivo* retroviral transfection to overexpress the prosurvival gene *Akt1* (encoding the Akt protein). Transplantation of five millions of MSCs overexpressing Akt into the ischemic rat myocardium had inhibited the process of ventricular remodeling by reducing intramyocardial inflammation, collagen deposition and myocardial hypertrophy, restoring 80%~90% of the lost myocardial volume, and completely normalizing systolic and diastolic ventricular function. MSCs carried with the *Akt1* gene had restored four-fold higher left ventricular volume *in vivo* transplantation than an equal number of MSCs transfected with the reporter gene *lacZ*FeN (Mangi et al, 2003). Akt might alter the secretion of a series of cytokines and growth factors (Gnecchi, 2005, 2006). MSCs overexpressing Akt have dramatically repaired the infarcted myocardium and improved cardiac function despite infrequent cellular fusion or transdifferentiation (Noiseux et al, 2006).

In addition, Zhang and colleagues had transfected MSCs with retrovirus to overexpress endothelium nitric oxide synthetase (eNOS). They reported that compared with vector transfected MSCs, *eNOS*-MSCs could significantly promote neovascularization onto the electrospun tubular scaffolds. Furthermore, transplantaion of MSCs overexpressing cell chemokine receptor-1 (CCR-1) transfected by retrovirus into AMI animal models could markedly promote cell homing to the ischemic myocardium and become involved in the repair process (Huang et al, 2007).

6.4 Lentivirus and Pacemaker Current Gene

There are some reports on transfection of MSCs with lentivirus vectors. Although the transfection efficiency is relatively high and the transfection procedure does not change the properties of stem cells, a low virual titration could lead to cytotoxicity under some conditions.

Hyperpolarization-activated cyclic-nucleotide-modulated (HCN) channel gene family is a key player in pacing, which encodes pacemaker current If. Plasmid pcDNA3-*hHCN2* by lipofectin could be successfully transfected by lentivirus into rat MSCs with If recorded by whole-cell patch clamp technique (Li et al, 2006). Genetically modified human MSCs can express functional HCN2 channels *in vitro* and *in vivo*, mimicking over expression of *HCN2* genes in cardiac myocytes (Potapova et al, 2004). Transfected human MSCs influenced the beating rate *in vitro* when plated onto a localized region of a coverslip and overlaid with neonatal rat ventricular myocytes. The coculture beating rate was increased from 93±16 bpm to 161±4 bpm. When investigators subepicardialy injected a million human MSCs transfected with *mHCN2* gene in the left ventricular wall of a canine *in situ*, during sinus arrest, 5 out of 6 animals developed spontaneous ventricular rhythms of left-sided origin (rate=61±5 bpm). The human MSCs transfected with HCN have the ablility to develop a biological pacemaker in the heart. Zhou YF and collaborators had also transfected MSCs with *HCN2* genes by lentivirus (Zhou, 2007). Transfected cells were overexpressing characteristic hHCN2 protein and the If-like current, increasing the spontaneous beating rate in the coculture system with cardiomyocytes. HIV1-based lentiviral vector (LentiV) for transgene delivery can integrate target genes into the host genome. This unique property makes lentivirus ideal for modifying MSCs, which allows persistent expression of transfected genes.

6.5 Conclusion

Since MSCs have pluripotent transdifferentiation properties and can easily be isolated and cultured *ex vivo*, they are regarded as an ideal candidate for gene therapy and engineering. Though it appears hopeful, a future for MSCs in gene therapy, should be regarded with caution until more research is available (Lu et al, 2007). Safety during the transfection processes is critical to investigators, because the efficiency of transduction by non-virus is much lower. Also, keeping a persistent and stable expression of target genes is also challenging. Gene modification of MSCs by viral or non-viral vectors *in vitro* can lead to overexpression of target genes, but the expression can be transient and unstable.

In summary, due to their biological characteristics, research into MSCs as host cells for gene therapy is gradually becoming novel. The combination of gene transfection with pluripotent transdifferentiation will lead to a broad range of clinical applications. With further investigation of the properties of MSCs, gene therapy mediated by MSCs may be able to conquer many human diseases.

References

Bao C, Guo J, Lin G, Hu M, Hu Z (2007) TNFR gene-modified mesenchymal stem cells attenuate inflammation and cardiac dysfunction following MI. Scand Cardiovasc J, 24:1-7

Gao F, He T, Wang H, Yu S, Yi D, Liu W, Cai Z (2007) A promising strategy for the treatment of ischemic heart disease: Mesenchymal stem cell-mediated vascular endothelial growth factor gene transfer in rats. Can J Cardiol, 23(11):891-898

Gnecchi M, He H, Liang OD, Melo LG, Morello F, Mu H, Noiseux N, Zhang L, Pratt RE, Ingwall JS, Dzau VJ (2005) Paracrine action accounts for marked protection of ischemic heart by Akt-modified mesenchymal stem cells. Nat Med,11(4):367-368

Gnecchi M, He H, Noiseux N, Liang OD, Zhang L, Morello F, Mu H, Melo LG, Pratt RE, Ingwall JS, Dzau VJ (2006) Evidence supporting paracrine hypothesis for Akt-modified mesenchymal stem cell-mediated cardiac protection and functional improvement. FASEB J, 20(6):661-669

Guan SY, Zeng QT, Chen B, Lang MJ (2006) Transplantation of allogenetic mesenchymal stem cells transfected with vascular endothelial growth factor gene into rat infarcted myocardium. Acta Med Univ Sci Tech Huazhong, 35(3):305-309

Guo YT, Li XY (2003) The expression of *SERCa-2* gene transfer into bone marrow msenchymal stem cells of the rats. Chin J Molecular Cardiology, 4(3):155-159

Huang J, Guo J, Ni A, Deb A, Zhang L, Prattre R, Dzau VJ (2007) Genetically modified mesenchymal stem cells (MSCs) overexpressing chemokine receptor CCR1 improves cellular engraftment and tissue repair of ischemic myocardium. Circulation, 116: II_132

Li HL, Li HW, Xing FY, Sun XG, Deng YB, Zhang XM, Jiang Y, Li SN (2003) Construction of recombinant adenovirus expressing BDNF and its expression in expanded rat mesenchymal stem cells *in vitro*. Chin J Pathophysiology, 19(4): 438-442

Li HX, Yang XJ, Zhao X, Jiang B, Cheng XJ, Chen T, Han LH, Song JP, Liu ZH, Jiang WP (2006) Pacemaker current gene expression of rat mesenchymal stem cells and identification of mesenchymal stem cells expressing human pacemaker current gene(*hHCN2*). Zhonghua Xin Xue Guan Bing Za Zhi, 34(10):917-921

Li W, Ma N, Ong LL, Nesselmann C, Klopsch C, Ladilov Y, Furlani D, Piechaczek C, Moebius JM, Ltzow K, Lendlein A, Stamm C, Li RK, Steinhoff G (2007) *Bcl-2* engineered MSCs inhibited apoptosis and improved heart function. Stem Cells, 25(8): 2118-2127

Lu LL, Zhao HY, Zhao CL, Sun XH, Duan CL, Yang H (2007) Comparison in techniques of gene transfection for bone marrow derived mesenchymal stem cells. J Clin Rehabilitative Tissue Engineering Res, 11(3):471-474

Mangi AA, Noiseux N, Kong D, He H, Rezvani M, Ingwall JS, Dzau VJ (2003) Mesenchymal stem cells modified with Akt prevent remodeling and restore performance of infarcted hearts. Nat Med, 9(9):1195-1201

Matsumoto R, Omura T, Yoshiyama M, Hayashi T, Inamoto S, Koh KR, Ohta K, Izumi Y, Nakamura Y, Akioka K, Kitaura Y, Takeuchi K, Yoshikawa J (2005) Vascular endothelial growth factor-expressing mesenchymal stem cell transplantation for the treatment of acute myocardial infarction. Arterioscler Thromb Vasc Biol, 25(6):1168-1173

McMahon JM, Conroy S, Lyons M, Greiser U, O'shea C, Strappe P, Howard L, Murphy M, Barry F, O'Brien T (2006) Gene transfer into rat mesenchymal stem cells: a comparative study of viral and nonviral vectors. Stem Cells Dev, 15(1):87-96

Noiseux N, Gnecchi M, Lopez-Ilasaca M, Zhang L, Solomon SD, Deb A, Dzau VJ, Pratt RE (2006) Mesenchymal stem cells overexpressing Akt dramatically repair infarcted myocardium and improve cardiac function despite infrequent cellular fusion or differentiation. Mol Ther, 14(6):840-850

Potapova I, Plotnikov A, Lu Z, Danilo P Jr, Valiunas V, Qu J, Doronin S, Zuckerman J, Shlapakova IN, Gao J, Pan Z, Herron AJ, Robinson RB, Brink PR, Rosen MR, Cohen IS (2004) Human mesenchymal stem cells as a gene delivery system to create cardiac pacemakers. Circ Res, 94(7):952-959

Sun L, Cui M, Wang Z, Feng X, Mao J, Chen P, Kangtao M, Chen F, Zhou C (2007) Mesenchymal stem cells modified with angiopoietin-1 improve remodeling in a rat model of acute myocardial infarction. Biochem Biophys Res Commun, 357(3):779-784

Yang J, Zhou W, Zheng W, Ma Y, Lin L, Tang T, Liu J, Yu J, Zhou X, Hu J (2007) Effects of myocardial transplantation of marrow mesenchymal stem cells transfected with vascular endothelial growth factor for the improvement of heart function and angiogenesis after myocardial infarction Cardiology,107(1):17-29

Zheng QW, Dong XX, Peng Y, Dong WH, Liang ZP, He HH, Zhou P, Liu JB (2005) Retroviral-mediated high efficient expression of target gene in expanded rat mesenchymal stem cells. Chin J Modern Med, 15(22):3424-3431

Zhou WW, Hu JG, Yang JF, Lin L, Zhou XM, Tang T (2006) Angiogenic effect of bone marrow mesenchymal stem cells transfected with human VEGF gene on myocardial infarcts in rats. Zhong Nan Da Xue Xue Bao Yi Xue Ban, 31(5):763-766, 771

Zhou YF, Yang XJ, Li HX, Han LH, Jiang WP (2007) Mesenchymal stem cells transfected with HCN2 genes by LentiV can be modified to be cardiac pacemaker cells. Med Hypotheses, 69(5):1093-1097

7

Feasibility of MSCs Transplantaion

Shaoping Wang[1]

[1]Second Affiliated Hospital, Zhejiang University College of Medicine, Hangzhou, China
E-mail: wang_shaoping@hotmail.com

Abstract: A number of practical problems need to be addressed before any form of cell therapy can be widely applied in patients with multiple diseases. The choice of cell type is one considered elsewhere in this issue; others include the question of ethics, the mode of delivery of cells, the timing of any treatment and perhaps above all the safety of the patient. Here we review the progress in various of these practical problems in order to explain how we have arrived at the conclusion that the clinical science has progressed to a stage where MSCs can be safely and appropriately applied to treat patients with cardiovascular diseases.

The complex moral and ethical debates surrounding the definition of the origins of human life, together with conflicting current and proposed legislation, are hindering the course of research into the therapeutic utilization of human embryonic stem cells (ESCs) (Moore et al, 2006; Dawson et al, 2003). However, adult stem cells, free from many of the ethical and legal concerns attached to ESCs, offer great promise for the advancement of medicine. Several lines of enquiry suggest the plausibility of using stem cell therapy for the treatment of cardiovascular diseases in adults. These alternative sources may alleviate the need to resolve the debates on stem cells before further therapeutic benefits of stem cell transplantation can be realized.

Nevertheless, a substantial amount of basic, translational, and clinical research will be required to properly assess such approaches to adult stem cell usage. There are still many essential ethical issues to be addressed (Sugarman, 2007). Here we discuss some of the key ethical considerations regarding research involving bone marrow-derived mesenchymal stem cell (MSC) therapy in cardiovascular diseases.

7.1 General Ethical Considerations

There are a series of ethical considerations that must be taken into account in making the transition from bench to bedside, safety, the possibility of benefits, the experimental designs and informed consent. Careful consideration must firstly be taken regarding the safety of these proposed interventions before they are introduced to human beings. The ethical obligation of protecting human safety is central to a code of ethics, both for basic research and clinical healthcare. In large part, the data necessary to make such a determination will be derived from animal experiments, as well as previous related human research, and the medical condition of potential human subjects. These data need to be considered in the context of therapeutic alternatives when considering a new intervention. If safety can be reasonably ensured, then the answer to these important scientific questions should be determined. By promoting the goals of safety and using a sound research design, the therapeutic benefits can be ascertained. Finally, any potential research subjects must be in a position to give informed consent.

7.2 Safety Issues

The risk of infectious disease transmission from donor to recipient is common to all types of tissue and organ transplantation. Thus, under most conditions, the risks associated with the transmission of infections by MSCs transplantation must be characterized on the basis of previous research concerning other types of tissue donation. Screening is essential to protect the recipients from infectious agents, but sometimes emergent infectious diseases escaping the detection have posed a problem. Currently, transplantation of autologous MSCs is much more popular than an allogenic strategy, which avoids the transmission of infectious diseases from donor to recipient. However, other types of infection from micro-organisms are involved in this situation. Medical hygiene is important during MSCs isolation, expansion, storage and transfer from the laboratory to the patient. In addition, serum is commonly used as a supplement to MSCs culture medium. The most widely used animal serum is fetal bovine serum. Because serum is an ill-defined component and a xenologous protein, serum-free cell culture media should be developed as an alternative to the use of animal serum. Superior manufacturing practices and quality control procedures need to be established for the isolation of MSCs that will potentially be used for future cell therapies.

Adult stem cells are those which show long-term replicative potential, together with the capacity for self-renewal and multi-lineage differentiation. These stem cell properties are tightly regulated in normal development, yet their alteration may be a critical issue for tumorogenesis. This concept has arisen from the striking degree of similarity noted between somatic stem cells and cancer cells, including the fundamental ability of self-renewal and differentiation. Given these strikingly identical properties, it has been proposed that cancers are caused by transforming mutations occurring in tissue-specific stem cells (Martnez-Climent et al, 2006). Also, recent experiments showing that transplanted adult hematopoietic stem cells (HSCs) can fuse with liver cells in the mouse are also cause for concern (Wang et al, 2003; Vassilopoulos et al, 2003). Fusion events that result in tetraploidy may produce cells that are inherently unstable and prone to chromosome loss and uncontrolled growth, thus producing tumors in the recipients. Although little data has been collected, clinical research so far has disclosed that tumors can form in MSC transplantation, making the practice of long-term follow-up a necessity.

Recently, a number of early-phase clinical studies with small numbers of patients have addressed the question of arrhythmogenosis in cardiac cell transplantation. Unlike skeletal myoblast transplantation, in which two of the five recruited patients experienced ventricular tachycardia (VT) in the immediate postoperative period (Pagani et al, 2003), most studies have demonstrated that MSC transplantation had a lesser proarrhythmia effect (Miyoshi et al, 2007). MSCs can express connexin 43 and form a gap junction among MSCs, as well as between MSCs and host cardiomyocytes (Pijnappels et al, 2006). However, we can not exclude the possibility of arrhythmogensis. Firstly, the conduction velocity in the MSCs is less than that of an intact human heart. The lower gap junction size and density, and less developed ionic channel machinery may result in slower conduction velocities and may become a potential substrate for reentrant arrhythmias (Chang et al, 2006). Secondly, it has been demonstrated that MSCs injection in the swine myocardium could increase sympathetic nerve density throughout the ventricles (Pak et al, 2003). Thus, although an increase of sympathetic innervation could increase contractility and the ejection fraction of the treated ventricles, it might also induce ventricular arrhythmias by increasing dispersion of repolarized cells and trigger arrhythmias, particularly in a damaged ventricle with abnormal ion channel activity caused by electrical remodeling. Thirdly, tissue injury could be responsible for arrhythmogenesis after intramyocardial MSC injection. Local injection also induces a highly uneven distribution of cells, at least soon after injection, which increases electrophysiological heterogeneity.

There may be some other potential safety issues concerning MSCs, such as the loss of transplanted cells, stent restenosis, microthrombosis (Kang et al, 2004; Vulliet et al, 2004), and viral infection, especially with viral transfected MSCs. In a word, from the viewpoint of ethics, the issue of safety is paramount. Well-designed experiments and rigorous long-term follow-up are critically important when we assess the safety of a new methodology.

7.3 Informed Consent

Informed consent is now an established requirement for research with human subjects. Obtaining informed consent necessitates the need for the potential subject to have adequate decision making capabilities, and be competent at the time consent is being solicited. An adequate capacity to give consent includes the ability to take in new information, to process that information, to make a decision based on that information, and to be able to express the decision. In addition, relevant information needs to be disclosed in a manner that is understandable to the potential subject.

In considering stem cell therapy for cardiovascular disease, questions about the adequacy of decisions may arise if experimental interventions are intended to be given in the setting of acute cardiac events that may be associated with pain, anxiety, and psychological treatments. Thus, for research planned in these settings, it seems obligatory for investigators to set up a series of explicit protocols for evaluating whether patients can consider adequately and make decisions before signing the consent.

Fueled partly by disease-based activism, patients with severe pathology usually desire participation. The desire for access to clinical research can also make the informed consent process especially challenging. It has now been well documented that many patients enrolled in clinical research harbor a therapeutic misconception, in which they believe erroneously that the primary purpose of the research is to care for them as patients rather than to address a scientific problem. Similarly, a therapeutic misconception may be involved that patients believe erroneously that although treatment assignments in the trials are randomized, their specific assignment was optimally determined by their physician. Therefore, when patients request or demand participation in trials, special attention should be paid to clarifying the understanding of the patients in case of a therapeutic misconception.

7.4 Conclusion

Research on MSC therapies for cardiovascular disease is scientifically exciting. Although most of this research has challenging ethical concerns, it can be addressed by taking appropriate measures. For those engaged in this research and these ethical issues, four principles should be the primary concern of the investigators involved: autonomy, benefits, non-malfeasance and justice.

References

Chang MG, Tung L, Sekar RB, Chang CY, Cysyk J, Dong P, Marbn E, Abraham MR (2006) Proarrhythmic potential of mesenchymal stem cell transplantation revealed in an *in vitro* coculture model. Circulation, 113(15):1832-1841

Dawson L, Bateman-House AS, Mueller Agnew D, Bok H, Brock DW, Chakravarti A, Greene M, King PA, O'Brien SJ, Sachs DH, Schill KE, Siegel A, Solter D, Suter SM, Verfaillie CM, Walters LB, Gearhart JD, Faden RR (2003) Safety issues in cell-based intervention trials. Fertil Steril, 80(5):1077-1085

Kang HJ, Kim HS, Zhang SY, Park KW, Cho HJ, Koo BK, Kim YJ, Soo Lee D, Sohn DW, Han KS, Oh BH, Lee MM, Park YB (2004) Effects of intracoronary infusion of peripheral blood stem-cells mobilised with granulocyte-colony stimulating factor on left ventricular systolic function and restenosis after coronary stenting in myocardial infarction: the MAGIC cell randomised clinical trial. Lancet, 363(9411):751-756

Martnez-Climent JA, Andreu EJ, Prosper F (2006) Somatic stem cells and the origin of cancer Clin Transl Oncol, 8(9):647-663

Miyoshi S, Ikegami Y, Itabashi Y, Furuta A, Umezawa A, Ogawa S (2007) Cardiac cell therapy and arrhythmias. Circ J, 71(A):A45-A49

Moore KE, Mills JF, Thornton MM (2006) Alternative sources of adult stem cells: a possible solution to the embryonic stem cell debate. Gend Med, 3(3):161-168

Pagani FD, DerSimonian H, Zawadzka A, Wetzel K, Edge AS, Jacoby DB, Dinsmore JH, Wright S, Aretz TH, Eisen HJ, Aaronson KD (2003) Autologous skeletal myoblasts transplanted to ischemia-damaged myocardium in humans. Histological analysis of cell survival and differentiation J Am Coll Cardiol, 41(5):879-888

Pak HN, Qayyum M, Kim DT, Hamabe A, Miyauchi Y, Lill MC, Frantzen M, Takizawa K, Chen LS, Fishbein MC, Sharifi BG, Chen PS, Makkar R (2003) Mesenchymal stem cell injection induces cardiac nerve sprouting and increased tenascin expression in a swine model of myocardial infarction. J Cardiac Electrophysiol, 14(8):841-848

Pijnappels DA, Schalij MJ, van Tuyn J, Ypey DL, de Vries AA, van der Wall EE, van der Laarse A, Atsma DE (2006) Progressive increase in conduction velocity across human mesenchymal stem cells is mediated by enhanced electrical coupling. Cardiovasc Res, 72(2):282-291

Sugarman J (2007) Ethics and stem cell therapeutics for cardiovascular disease. Prog Cardiovasc Dis, 50(1):1-6

Vassilopoulos G, Wang PR, Russell DW (2003) Transplanted bone marrow regenerates liver by cell fusion. Nature, 422(6934):901-904

Vulliet PR, Greeley M, Halloran SM, MacDonald KA, Kittleson MD (2004) Intracoronary arterial injection of mesenchymal stromal cells and microinfarction in dogs. Lancet, 363 (9411):783-784

Wang X, Willenbring H, Akkari Y, Torimaru Y, Foster M, Al-Dhalimy M, Lagasse E, Finegold M, Olson S, Grompe M (2003) Cell fusion is the principal source of bone-marrow-derived hepatocytes Nature, 422(6934):897-901

8

Status and Expectation of MSCs Therapy

Shaoping Wang[1]

[1]Second Affiliated Hospital, Zhejiang University College of Medicine, Hangzhou, China
E-mail: wang_shaoping@hotmail.com

Abstract: MSCs therapy for cardiovascular diseases: beginning or end of the road? As our understanding of stem-cell behavior rapidly increases, more and more reports suggest that use of MSCs therapy will extend well beyond regenerative medicine in the near future. In this chapter, we also provide an outline of the rationale and status of stem-cell-based treatments for cardiovascular diseases, and we discuss prospects for clinical implementation and the factors crucial for maintaining momentum towards this goal.

Recently, China Multicenter Collaborative Studies of Cardiovascular Epidemiology (CMCSCE) has published findings to show that cardiovascular disease is the overwhelming cause of death for both men and women, with strokes accounting for over 40% of deaths in China (Liu, 2007). With rapid socioeconomic progress, coronary heart disease (CHD) and heart failure continue to be significant burdens on healthcare systems. Therefore, any new treatment modality that benefits patients suffering from heart failure has the potential to result in a dramatic improvement in health and substantial cost savings for the community.

8.1 Clinical Application and Outcomes

The possibility of using stem cell-based therapies for people suffering with acute myocardial infarction (AMI) or congestive heart failure (CHF) has captured the imagination of both the medical and public communities. Since early reports of animal models more than 10 years ago, the research field of stem cells has made enormous advances in moving toward clinically applicable treatment options. We are now standing at the dawn of a new therapeutic era.

At present a number of early clinical studies have been published. Abdel-Latif and colleagues had published a systematic review and meta-analysis of adult bone marrow-derived cells (BMCs) for cardiac repair (Abdel-Latif et al, 2007). They have summarized all the randomized, placebo-controlled trials and cohort studies of BMCs transplantation to treat ischemic heart disease (IHD) (Table 8.1). Eighteen studies (patients n=999) were eligible and included. BMCs transplantation improved left ventricular ejection fraction (LVEF) at 3.66% [95% confidence interval (CI), 1.93% to 5.40%; P=0.001], reduced 5.49% of infarcted scar size (95% CI, –9.10% to –1.88%; P=0.003), and decreased 4.80ml of left ventricular end-systolic volume (LVESV, 95% CI, –8.20 to –1.41ml; P=0.006). These results suggest that BMCs transplantation is associated with modest improvements in physiological and anatomic parameters in patients with both AMI and chronic ischemic heart disease (IHD), beyond conventional therapy. It seems that BMCs therapy is also safe. Hristov and coworkers have reviewed randomized placebo-controlled clinical studies, comparing the combination therapy of intracoronary autologous non-mobilized BMCs injection with standard medical therapy versus standard therapy alone in patients with AMI (Hristov et al, 2006). They have identified five randomized, controlled clinical trials, three of which were both placebo- and bone marrow aspirate-controlled. The overall effects on the change of LVEF from the results of baseline and follow-up was analyzed, which revealed a significant improvement (4.21%) in the BMCs-treated group as compared to the control group (95% CI, 0.21% to 8.22%; P=0.04). In contrast, the overall effects on LVEF did not reveal a significant difference between both groups in follow-up (P=0.16).

Table 8.1. Characteristics of studies included in the Meta-analysis

Authors	Study Design	Patient No.	Disease	Mean follow-up (months)	Cell Type	No. of Cells	Delivery Route	Time from PCI and/or MI to Transplantation (days*)	Ref.
Assmus	RCT	92	ICM	3	BMMNC CPC	$(205 \pm 110) \times 10^6$ $(22 \pm 11) \times 10^6$	IC	2348 ± 2318 2470 ± 2196	(Assmus et al, 2006)
Bartunek	Cohort	35	AMI	4	BMMNC($CD133^+$)	$(12.6 \pm 2.2) \times 10^6$	IC	11.6 ± 1.4	(Bartunek et al, 2005)
Chen	RCT	69	AMI	6	MSC	$(48\sim60) \times 10^9$	IC	18.4 ± 0.5	(Chen et al, 2004)
Erbs	RCT	26	ICM	3	CPC	$(69 \pm 14) \times 10^6$	IC	225 ± 87	(Erbs et al, 2005)
Ge	RCT	20	AMI	6	BMMNC	40×10^6	IC	1	(Huang et al, 2006)
Hendrikx	RCT	20	ICM	4	BMMNC	$(60.25 \pm 31) \times 10^6$	IM	217 ± 162	(Hendrikx et al, 2006)
Janssens	RCT	67	AMI	4	BMMNC	$(172 \pm 72) \times 10^6$	IC	1~2 (Rang)	(Janssens et al, 2006)
Kang	RCT	82	AMI/ICM	6	CPC	$(14 \pm 5) \times 10^8$	IC	7 ± 1 (AMI) 517 ± 525 (OMI)	(Kang et al, 2006)
Katritsis	Cohort	22	AMI/ICM	4	MSC and EPC	$(2\sim4) \times 10^6$	IC	224 ± 470	(Katritsis et al, 2005)
Lunde	RCT	100	AMI	6	BMMNC	$(87 \pm 47.7) \times 10^6$	IC	6 ± 1.3	(Lunde et al, 2006)
Meyer	RCT	60	AMI	18	BMMNC	$(24.6 \pm 9.4) \times 10^8$	IC	4.8 ± 1.3	(Meyer et al, 2006)
Mocini	Cohort	36	ICM	3	BMMNC	$(292 \pm 232) \times 10^6$	IM	NR	(Mocini et al, 2006)
Perin	Cohort	20	ICM	12	BMMNC	$(25.5 \pm 6.3) \times 10^6$	IM	NR	(Perin et al, 2004)
Ruan	RCT	20	AMI	6	BMC	NR	IC	1	(Ruan et al, 2005)
Schächinger	RCT	204	AMI	4	BMMNC	$(236 \pm 174) \times 10^6$	IC	4.3 ± 1.3	(Schächinger et al, 2006)
Strauer	Cohort	20	AMI	3	BMMNC	$(28 \pm 22) \times 10^6$	IC	8 ± 2	(Strauer et al, 2002)
Strauer	Cohort	36	ICM	3	BMMNC	90×10^6	IC	823.5 ± 945.5	(Strauer et al, 2005)
Li	RCT	70	AMI	6	CPC (PBSC)	$(72.5 \pm 73.3) \times 10^6$	IC	7 ± 5	(Li et al, 2006)

Abbreviations: AMI, acute myocardial infarction; BMC, bone marrow cell; BMMNC, bone marrow mononuclear cell; CPC, circulating progenitor cell; EPC, endothelial progenitor cell; IC, intracoronary injection; ICM, ischemic cardiomyopathy; IM, intramyocardial injection using electromechanical mapping system; MI, myocardial infarction; MSC, mesenchymal stem cell; NR, not reported; OMI, old myocardial infarction; PBSC, peripheral blood stem cells; * Values are given as mean SD unless otherwise specified.

Published clinical controlled trials of BMCs infusion appear to be safe and feasible for patients with AMI as a supportive treatment. This is largely based on the notion that no apparent side effects or complications (e.g. arrhythmias, increased ischemia with subsequent microembolism) have been reported. However, the studies remain controversial with respect to their effectiveness in improving the cardiac function. Compared with a randomized control group, the BOOST trial did not show any long-term benefits of BMCs infusion on left ventricular (LV) systolic function for patients with AMI, but suggested an acceleration of LVEF restoration at 18 months follow-up (Wollert et al, 2004; Meyer et al, 2006). As indicated above, both reviews of meta-analysis revealed that cell therapy offered only marginal improvement in LVEF, 3.66% in the former and 4.21% in the latter. The question of whether a small increase in LVEF is of clinical significance is an important issue. It should be stressed that most of the treatments with an established life-saving effect on AMI also provide moderate yet clinically meaningful increases of LVEF. Therefore, considering the increases of LVEF in the follow-up, BMC transplantation may be a safe and beneficial procedure to supplementally treat IHD. Since the functional improvement observed with these trials is relatively moderate and the studies are heterogeneous in design, further efforts aiming at double-blind, randomized and placebo-controlled multi-center trials are required, with an appropriate criterion in patients enrolled (Boyle et al, 2006).

8.2 Mechanism of Therapeutic Effects

One of the major obstacles to the progress of large-scale clinical trials for stem cell therapy is the ongoing debate regarding the mechanism of the therapeutic effects of cardiac repairing. The traditional notion providing the primary motivation to stem cell therapy is that stem cells transplantaion would repair the damaged myocardium via transdifferentiating and by promoting myocardial regeneration (Orlic et al, 2001). However, the results from recent studies have led to a novel recognition of the effect and its mechanisms, as shown in Fig. 8.1. Exogenous stem cells performed cell fusion with host cardiomyocytes (Nygren et al, 2004). Proliferation of endogenous cardiac precursors or stem cells (CPC/CSC) might be promoted by exogenous engrafted cells mediated by neovascularization (Kocher et al, 2001; Schuster et al, 2004) or paracrine effects (Gnecchi et al, 2005). Cellular therapy may contribute to the restoration of stem cell niches, facilitating the endogenous healing processes (Moore and Lemischka, 2006). Some investigators suggest that the therapeutic effects of stem cells are mediated by adjusting mechanical properties to strengthen the MI scar (Wang et al, 2006) or improving the electrical viability of the injured heart (Mills et al, 2007), thereby preventing deterioration in cardiac function. This ongoing debate about the mechanisms of stem cell therapy

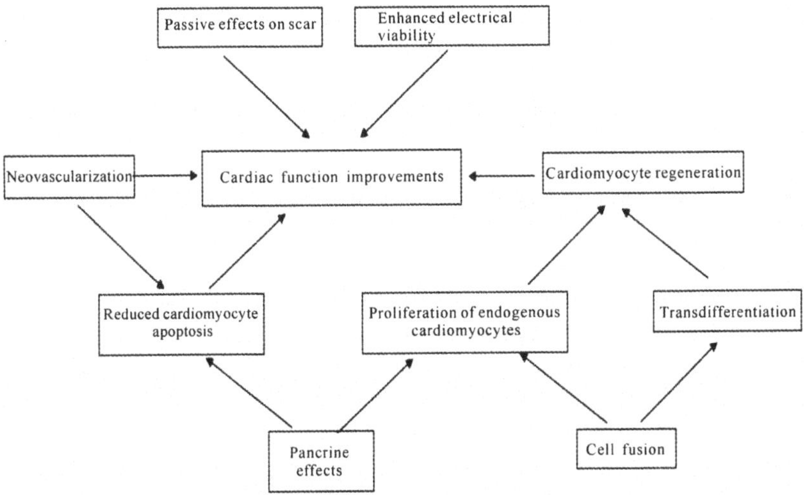

Fig. 8.1. Possible mechanisms for successful cardiac repair by stem cells

might fuel the case for slowing the pace of clinical trials. We should not pursue transplantation in patients until we have drawn a thorough conclusion from the outcomes *in vitro* and *in vivo* of cell therapy in animal models. However, we should objectively assess the results from a multitude of clinical studies and animal experiements and further clarify some issues important to the issue before this therapy is widely utilized in clinical practice.

8.3 Expectations with MSCs Therapy

When assessing the possibility of adopting a new treatment in clinical practice, rigorous scientific and ethical standards must be followed. Stem cell therapy has presented us with a number of unique challenges, not only the optimal cell type, but also the delivery pathway. These questions can be addressed only by objectively designed clinical trials. Our understanding of the exact mechanisms by which stem cells exert their beneficial effects on cardiac function has evolved substantially, initially assuming transdifferentiation as the only mode for its therapeutic effects, and subsequently extending to other possibilities, including strengthening cardiac scar area and paracrine effects. Importantly, we propose that all of these features may be integrated into the repairing mechanism, which involves restoring endogenous stem cell niches.

Despite an incomplete understanding of the exact mechanism, many preclinical and clinical studies have consistently demonstrated the beneficial effects on the cardiac function as mentioned above. These beneficial findings cannot be ignored, and the ongoing clinical studies are aimed at a better understanding of the molecular underpinnings, because these functional improvements may be translated into clinical benefits for patients. These ethical and logistic issues, not encountered by most previous trials dealing with medications or devices, may appear daunting. However, despite the difficulties for stem cell research, basic tenets should be adopted for clinical observations.

- Safety is paramount for patients.
- Deprivation of a novel therapy must be considered against the inherent risk in testing it.

The overwhelming issue is the safety of the novel therapy before its adoption in clinical practice. "To do no harm" is, as always, our overriding concern. But how many data regarding safety are enough to justify advancing to the next stage of clinical investigation? Autologous stem cell therapy begins with the premise that cellular repair occurs naturally in the human body and that transplantation procedure should be safe. Actually, numerous animal studies have identified that this is the case, with no adverse effects of cellular therapy for cardiac repair being observed, which has served as the platform for the inception of human studies. Nearly 1,000 patients have been tested, and the totality of evidence from these studies supports the safety of cell therapy (Table 8.1). Large-scale and well-designed studies with clinical end points are required to further confirm the conclusion.

The risk of exposing patients to possible adverse outcomes by a new treatment must be weighed against the risk of depriving all patients of a new and possibly effective treatment to alleviate suffering or prolong life. There is now sufficient preclinical and clinical data to warrant larger randomized controlled trials for assessing stem cell therapy. The argument that these trials should be delayed until mechanisms are completely understood is unnecessary, and will deprive a large number of patients of therapeutic approaches that may improve their clinical outcome. Only clinical investigation can lead to the optimization of stem cell therapy with recognition of the best type of cell and the best delivery method for patients.

Another compelling argument for initiating clinical research is that the results of these investigations always provide pivotal insights, which push new methods forward. This concept is illustrated by several examples in cardiovascular medicine. ACE inhibitors (Faggiotto and Paoletti, 1999) and statins (Calabr and Yeh, 2005), widely used drugs with solid mechanistic underpinning to support their use, were both appreciated after entry into clinical practice and found to have additional pharmacological effects that extended beyond initial expectations. This would imply that clinical trials and basic experiments work in parallel in guiding the clinical application.

Another example is the development history of percutaneous transluminal coronary angioplasty (PTCA). In 1977, pioneer Andreas Grüntzig published results from an experiment on 8 dogs (Grüntzig and Schneider, 1977), then progressed to human postmortem observations and then to human clinical trials, publishing his first series concerning 5 patients only 1 year later (Grüntzig et al, 1978). The first study of 50 patients followed in 1979 (Grüntzig, 1979). This translational research program introduced PTCA as a new clinical treatment, but was not free from serious complications. Soon the problem of restenosis, the Achilles heel of PTCA, was appreciated, prompting substantial new basic research and the development of the coronary artery stent, which reduced but did not eliminate the incidence of restenosis. As is well known, drug-eluting stents (DES) that nearly eliminate restenosis have been developed. Before the publication of this seminal article (Morice et al, 2002), safety and feasibility data had been published on less than 100 patients (Sousa et al, 2001), substantially less than the number enrolled in preliminary stem cell trials.

Currently, a number of clinical trials on stem cell therapy for cardiac repair are Phase I or II trials rather than large Phase III trials, some of which continue to be nonrandomized. Clinical studies of stem cell therapy should use rigorous trial designs and intrinsic safeguard mechanisms. In this regard, they should be prospective, double-blind studies with randomization on a background of best conventional therapy. Clinical trials should be designed to go beyond surrogate end points, to detect differences in relevant clinical end points such as survival, hospitalization or reinfarction. Furthermore, future studies should be designed not only to assess safety and efficacy, but gain further insight into the therapeutic mechanism of stem cells, for example, stem cells after radiation preconditioning , which have no potential for proliferation but remain important to the paracrine system.

In summary, the transition from preliminary studies to randomized controlled trials will demonstrate the efficacy and the safety of these therapies, thereby adopting them in clinical practice. We anticipate the coming of that day.

References

Abdel-Latif A, Bolli R, Tleyjeh IM, Montori VM, Perin EC, Hornung CA, Zuba-Surma EK, Al-Mallah M, Dawn B (2007) Adult bone marrow-derived cells for cardiac repair: a systematic review and meta-analysis. Arch Intern Med, 167(10):989-997

Assmus B, Honold J, Schächinger V, Britten MB, Fischer-Rasokat U, Lehmann R, Teupe C, Pistorius K, Martin H, Abolmaali ND, Tonn T, Dimmeler S, Zeiher AM (2006) Transcoronary transplantation of progenitor cells after myocardial infarction. N Engl J Med, 355(12):1222-1232

Bartunek J, Vanderheyden M, Vandekerckhove B, Mansour S, De Bruyne B, De Bondt P, Van Haute I, Lootens N, Heyndrickx G, Wijns W (2005) Intracoronary injection of CD133 positive enriched bone marrow progenitor cells promotes cardiac recovery after recent myocardial infarction: feasibility and safety. Circulation, 112(9 Suppl):I178-I183

Boyle AJ, Schulman SP, Hare JM, Oettgen P (2006) Is stem cell therapy ready for patients? Stem cell therapy for cardiac repair: ready for the next step. Circulation, 114(4):339-352

Calabr P, Yeh ET (2005) The pleiotropic effects of statins. Curr Opin Cardiol, 20(6): 541-546

Chen SL, Fang WW, Ye F, Liu YH, Qian J, Shan SJ, Zhang JJ, Chunhua RZ, Liao LM, Lin S, Sun JP (2004) Effect on left ventricular function of intracoronary transplantation of autologous bone marrow mesenchymal stem cell in patients with acute myocardial infarction. Am J Cardiol, 94(1):92-95

Erbs S, Linke A, Adams V, Lenk K, Thiele H, Diederich KW, Emmrich F, Kluge R, Kendziorra K, Sabri O, Schuler G, Hambrecht R (2005) Transplantation of blood-derived progenitor cells after recanalization of chronic coronary artery occlusion: first randomized and placebo-controlled study Circ Res, 97(8):756-762

Faggiotto A, Paoletti R (1999) State-of-the-Art lecture. Statins and blockers of the renin-angiotensin system: vascular protection beyond their primary mode of action. Hypertension, 34:987-996

Gnecchi M, He H, Liang OD, Melo LG, Morello F, Mu H, Noiseux N, Zhang L, Pratt RE, Ingwall JS, Dzau VJ (2005) Paracrine action accounts for marked protection of ischemic heart by Akt-modified mesenchymal stem cells. Nat Med,11:367-368

Grüntzig A, Schneider HJ (1977) The percutaneous dilatation of chronic coronary stenoses-experiments and morphology. Schweiz Med Wochenschr, 107(44): 1588

Grüntzig A (1978) Transluminal dilatation of coronary artery stenosis. Lancet, 311:263

Grüntzig AR, Senning A, Siegenthaler WE (1979) Nonoperative dilatation of coronary-artery stenosis: percutaneous transluminal coronary angioplasty. N Engl J Med, 301:61-68

Hendrikx M, Hensen K, Clijsters C, Jongen H, Koninckx R, Bijnens E, Ingels M, Jacobs A, Geukens R, Dendale P, Vijgen J, Dilling D, Steels P, Mees U, Rummens JL (2006) Recovery of regional but not global contractile function by the direct intramyocardial autologous bone marrow transplantation: results from a randomized controlled clinical trial. Circulation, 114(1 Suppl):I101-107

Hristov M, Heussen N, Schober A, Weber C (2006) Intracoronary infusion of autologous bone marrow cells and left ventricular function after acute myocardial infarction: a meta-analysis. J Cell Mol Med, 10(3):727-733

Huang RC, Yao K, Zou YZ, Ge L, Qian JY, Yang J, Yang S, Niu YH, Li YL, Zhang YQ, Zhang F, Xu SK, Zhang SH, Sun AJ, Ge JB (2006) Long term follow-up on emergent intracoronary autologous bone marrow mononuclear cell transplantation for acute inferior-wall myocardial infarction. Chin J Med, 86(16):1107-1110

Janssens S, Dubois C, Bogaert J, Theunissen K, Deroose C, Desmet W, Kalantzi M, Herbots L, Sinnaeve P, Dens J, Maertens J, Rademakers F, Dymarkowski S, Gheysens O, Van Cleemput J, Bormans G, Nuyts J, Belmans A, Mortelmans L, Boogaerts M, Van de Werf F (2006) Autologous bone marrow-derived stem-cell transfer in patients with ST-segment elevation myocardial infarction: double-blind, randomised controlled trial. Lancet, 367(9505):113-121

Kang WJ, Kang HJ, Kim HS, Chung JK, Lee MC, Lee DS (2006) Tissue distribution of 18F-FDG-labeled peripheral hematopoietic stem cells after intracoronary administration in patients with myocardial infarction. J Nucl Med, 47(8):1295-1301

Katritsis DG, Sotiropoulou PA, Karvouni E, Karabinos I, Korovesis S, Perez SA, Voridis EM, Papamichail M (2005) Transcoronary transplantation of autologous mesenchymal stem cells and endothelial progenitors into infarcted human myocardium. Catheter Cardiovasc Interv Jul, 65(3):321-329

Kocher AA, Schuster MD, Szabolcs MJ, Takuma S, Burkhoff D, Wang J, Homma S, Edwards NM, Itescu S (2001) Neovascularization of ischemic myocardium by human bone-marrow-derived angioblasts prevents cardiomyocyte apoptosis, reduces remodeling and improves cardiac function. Nat Med, 7(4):430-436

Li ZQ, Zhang M, Jin YZ, Zhang WW, Liu Y, Yuan L, Cui LJ, Liu XZ, Yu X, Hu TS (2006) Safety and efficacy of intracoronary transplantation of G-CSF mobilized autologous peripheral blood stem cells in patients with acute myocardial infarction. Zhonghua Xin Xue Guan Bing Za Zhi, 34(2):99-102

Liu L (2007) Cardiovascular disease in China. Biochem Cell Biol, 85:157-163

Lunde K, Solheim S, Aakhus S, Arnesen H, Abdelnoor M, Egeland T, Endresen K, Ilebekk A, Mangschau A, Fjeld JG, Smith HJ, Taraldsrud E, Grgaard HK, Bjrnerheim R, Brekke M, Mller C, Hopp E, Ragnarsson A, Brinchmann JE, Forfang K (2006) Intracoronary injection of mononuclear bone marrow cells in acute myocardial infarction. N Engl J Med, 355(12):1199-1209

Meyer GP, Wollert KC, Lotz J, Steffens J, Lippolt P, Fichtner S, Hecker H, Schaefer A, Arseniev L, Hertenstein B, Ganser A, Drexler H (2006) Intracoronary bone marrow cell transfer after myocardial infarction: eighteen months' follow-up data from the randomized, controlled BOOST (BOne marrOw transfer to enhance ST-elevation infarct regeneration) trial. Circulation, 113(10):1287-1294

Mills WR, Mal N, Kiedrowski MJ, Unger R, Forudi F, Popovic ZB, Penn MS, Laurita KR (2007) Stem cell therapy enhances electrical viability in myocardial infarction. J Mol Cell Cardiol, 42(2):304-314

Mocini D, Staibano M, Mele L, Giannantoni P, Menichella G, Colivicchi F, Sordini P, Salera P, Tubaro M, Santini M (2006) Autologous bone marrow mononuclear cell transplantation in patients undergoing coronary artery bypass grafting. Am Heart J, 151(1):192-197

Moore KA, Lemischka IR (2006) Stem cells and their niches. Science, 311:1880-1885

Morice MC, Serruys PW, Sousa JE, Fajadet J, Ban Hayashi E, Perin M, Colombo A, Schuler G, Barragan P, Guagliumi G, Molnr F, Falotico R; RAVEL Study Group (2002) Randomized study with the sirolimus-coated bx velocity balloon-expandable stent in the treatment of patients with de novo native coronary artery lesions. A randomized comparison of a sirolimuseluting stent with a standard stent for coronary revascularization. N Engl J Med, 346:1773-1780

Nygren JM, Jovinge S, Breitbach M, Swn P, Rll W, Hescheler J, Taneera J, Fleischmann BK, Jacobsen SE (2004) Bone marrow-derived hematopoietic cells generate cardiomyocytes at a low frequency through cell fusion, but not trans-differentiation. Nat Med,10: 494-501

Orlic D, Kajstura J, Chimenti S, Jakoniuk I, Anderson SM, Li B, Pickel J, McKay R, Nadal-Ginard B, Bodine DM, Leri A, Anversa P (2001) Bone marrow cells regenerate infarcted myocardium. Nature, 410:701-705

Perin EC, Dohmann HF, Borojevic R, Silva SA, Sousa AL, Silva GV, Mesquita CT, Belm L, Vaughn WK, Rangel FO, Assad JA, Carvalho AC, Branco RV, Rossi MI, Dohmann HJ, Willerson JT (2004) Improved exercise capacity and ischemia 6 and 12 months after transendocardial injection of autologous bone marrow mononuclear cells for ischemic cardiomyopathy. Circulation, 110(11 Suppl 1):II213-218

Ruan W, Pan CZ, Huang GQ, Li YL, Ge JB, Shu XH (2005) Assessment of left ventricular segmental function after autologous bone marrow stem cells transplantation in patients with acute myocardial infarction by tissue tracking and strain imaging. Chin Med J (Engl),118(14):1175-1181

Schächinger V, Erbs S, Elssser A, Haberbosch W, Hambrecht R, Hlschermann H, Yu J, Corti R, Mathey DG, Hamm CW, Sselbeck T, Assmus B, Tonn T, Dimmeler S, Zeiher AM; REPAIR-AMI Investigators (2006) Intracoronary bone marrow-derived progenitor cells in acute myocardial infarction. N Engl J Med, 355(12):1210-1221

Schuster MD, Kocher AA, Seki T, Martens TP, Xiang G, Homma S, Itescu S (2004) Myocardial neovascularization by bone marrow angioblasts results in cardiomyocyte regeneration. Am J Physiol Heart Circ Physiol, 287(2):H525-532

Sousa JE, Costa MA, Abizaid AC, Rensing BJ, Abizaid AS, Tanajura LF, Kozuma K, Van Langenhove G, Sousa AG, Falotico R, Jaeger J, Popma JJ, Serruys PW (2001) Sustained suppression of neointimal proliferation by sirolimus-eluting stents: one-year angiographic and intravascular ultrasound follow-up. Circulation, 104(17):2007-2011

Strauer BE, Brehm M, Zeus T, Kstering M, Hernandez A, Sorg RV, Kgler G, Wernet P (2002) Repair of infarcted myocardium by autologous intracoronary mononuclear bone marrow cell transplantation in humans. Circulation, 106(15):1913-1918

Strauer BE, Brehm M, Zeus T, Bartsch T, Schannwell C, Antke C, Sorg RV, Kgler G, Wernet P, Mller HW, Kstering M (2005) Regeneration of human infarcted heart muscle by intracoronary autologous bone marrow cell transplantation in chronic coronary artery disease: the IACT Study. J Am Coll Cardiol, 46(9):1651-1658

Wang JA, Luo RH, Zhang X, Xie XJ, Hu XY, He AN, Chen J, Li JH (2006) Bone marrow mesenchymal stem cell transplantation combined with perindopril treatment attenuates infarction remodelling in a rat model of acute myocardial infarction. J Zhejiang Univ Sci B, 7(8):641-647

Wollert KC, Meyer GP, Lotz J, Ringes-Lichtenberg S, Lippolt P, Breidenbach C, Fichtner S, Korte T, Hornig B, Messinger D, Arseniev L, Hertenstein B, Ganser A, Drexler H (2004) Intracoronary autologous bone-marrow cell transfer after myocardial infarction: the BOOST randomised controlled clinical trial. Lancet, 364(9429): 141-148

Index

The manufacturer's authorised representative in the EU is Springer Nature Customer Service Centre GmbH, Europaplatz 3, 69115 Heidelberg, Germany. If you have any concerns regarding our products, please contact ProductSafety@springernature.com

Printed and bound by CPI Group (UK) Ltd, Croydon, CR0 4YY
15/07/2026
02167645-0001